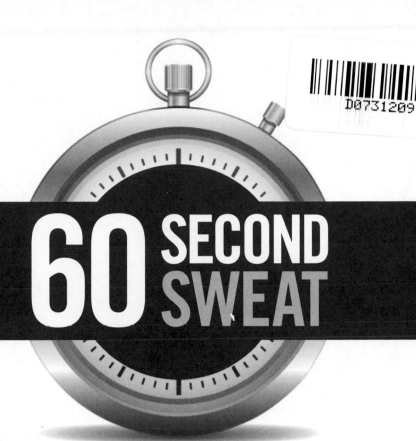

60 SECOND SWEAT

GET A ROCK-HARD BODY
1 MINUTE AT A TIME
WITH HIGH-INTENSITY INTERVAL
AND METABOLIC RESISTANCE TRAINING

PATRICK STRIET, CSCS
Owner of Live Fit Cincinnati

Reader's
digest

NEW YORK • MONTREAL

D0731209

A READER'S DIGEST BOOK

Copyright © 2017 Patrick Striet

All rights reserved. Unauthorized reproduction, in any manner, is prohibited.

Reader's Digest is a registered trademark of Trusted Media Brands, Inc.

All photos by Michael Bambino & Co. except for the following: page 7, courtesy of Katie O'Brien; page 11, courtesy of Nelson Lees; page 14, courtesy of Larry McGraw; page 21, courtesy of Donna Deye. Stopwatch image: Shutterstock.

Exercises in Part III are modeled by Patrick Striet and Stephanie Barber.

Library of Congress Cataloging-in-Publication Data

    Names: Striet, Patrick, author.
    Title: 60-second sweat : get a rock-hard body 1 minute at a time with
      high-intensity interval and metabolic resistance training / Patrick
      Striet, CSCS, owner of Live Fit Cincinnati.
    Description: New York : Reader's Digest / Trusted Media Brands, Inc. , [2016] | "A
      Reader's Digest Book"--T.p. verso. | Includes index.
    Identifiers: LCCN 2016027669 (print) | LCCN 2016038297 (ebook) | ISBN
      9781621453116 (paperback book : alk. paper) | ISBN 9781621453123 (epub)
    Subjects: LCSH: Physical fitness. | Exercise.
    Classification: LCC GV481 .S764 2016 (print) | LCC GV481 (ebook) | DDC
      613.7--dc23
    LC record available at https://lccn.loc.gov/2016027669

We are committed to both the quality of our products and the service we provide to our customers. We value your comments, so please feel free to contact us.

    Reader's Digest Trade Publishing
    44 South Broadway
    White Plains, NY 10601

For more Reader's Digest products and information, visit our website:

    www.rd.com (in the United States)
    www.readersdigest.ca (in Canada)

Printed in China

10 9 8 7 6 5 4 3 2 1

Contents

Introduction
Why the 60-Second Sweat?

There are—literally—thousands of fitness programs out there to choose from. So what makes the 60-Second Sweat different and why should you commit to it? It's a fair question.

Over the last 18 years "in the trenches" at my own fitness-training facility in Cincinnati, I've worked with hundreds of everyday men and women—working moms, college students, senior citizens, and middle-aged men (plus a few elite athletes). I have identified the barriers most people face when it comes to exercising consistently, as well as the shortcomings and drawbacks of the vast majority of fitness-training programs. I kept both of these at the forefront of my mind while crafting the 60-Second Sweat program.

Time—or lack thereof—is the biggest barrier most people face when it comes to adhering to a fitness program. We live in a fast-paced world, and the competing demands on our time have never been greater. Between 40-plus-hour workweeks, family responsibilities, and social commitments, many of us feel like there just isn't enough time to fit in consistent exercise . . . and with the unrealistic way most popular fitness regimens are organized, who could blame us?

Most mainstream fitness programs call for a 5- to 6-day commitment per week, with workouts ranging up to an hour (or more) in duration. What's more, most programs focus on 1 component of fitness in each workout. For example, you might do cardiovascular exercises for 45 minutes on Monday, Wednesday, and Friday, and then strength train for an hour on Tuesday, Thursday, and Saturday. Who has time for that? Not me . . . and probably not you either.

Beyond the unrealistic time commitment most modern fitness programs demand, most lack one or more of the following elements:

- **Progression:** To keep making progress, you need to make your workout more challenging over time.

- **Organization:** You want your workouts to flow, so it's easy to move from one exercise to the next and you're not overworking any particular muscles.

- **Safety:** If you get hurt, you can't train . . . and you can't make any gains in your level of fitness. Many popular workout programs include exercises which are, to put it mildly, completely inappropriate and increase the risk of injury.

- **Efficiency:** A workout that requires an unrealistic amount of time—or that includes unnecessary exercises—is one you won't follow. The exercises in your program should provide the greatest return on your time investment and should have a very logical purpose behind them.

- **Variety:** A workout that is boring is also one you won't follow. A good program should offer a nice mix of both progressive structure and variety over a period of time to keep you motivated.

Given all of the above, I took great care in developing this program to ensure the greatest "bang for your training buck." The 60-Second Sweat is progressive, organized, safe, efficient, and varied, while addressing every component of fitness in each workout.

Beyond that, the 60-Second Sweat is based on the most up-to-date, modern principles of exercise science, while also keeping in mind the typical chronic orthopedic issues most real-world adults face: cranky knees, aching backs, stiff shoulders, and sore necks. The 60-Second Sweat is not a generic, boring, machine-based circuit that members are given at the vast majority of commercial gyms: It is a balanced plan based on functional movements, designed to help us improve the way we use our bodies in everyday life—picking up groceries, running to catch a train, pushing a child in a swing. Think about how much time we spend sitting in our daily lives: We sit in the car to and from work, sit all day in front of a computer at work, and then sit on the couch when we get home. The last thing you need is to spend your workout sitting in a machine performing guided, stabilized exercises on a fixed plane. That's the very antithesis of functional movement, which will have the greatest carryover to your daily life.

The 60-Second Sweat can help you:

- **Lose weight:** Want to look better in a swimsuit, get back in your skinny jeans, or drop jaws at your upcoming high school reunion? By combining the recommendations and principles in the 60-Second Nutrition chapter with the 60-Second Sweat workouts, you'll be able to burn fat, drop pounds, retain and build lean muscle mass, and ultimately show off all the contour and tone in your body.

- **Feel better:** Tired of living with chronic aches and pains? Worried that you're feeling that twinge in your knee more often? If that's you, this is definitely your program. The balanced, comprehensive, and functional nature of the exercises in this program will leave you feeling as good as you have in years. Your joints will have more mobility, your back and core will be stronger and more stable, and your muscles will be looser. If you are sick of getting out of bed in the morning and feeling like the Tin Man, you'll love the 60-Second Sweat.

- **Improve your general fitness:** The progressive and comprehensive nature of this program can take your overall fitness to the next level. Do you work out sporadically? This program will give you the structure and incentive to step it up. Never worked out, or haven't worked out in years? The scalable nature of this program will allow you to take baby steps and progress safely without getting overwhelmed.

Whichever of the above goals applies to you—or if they all do—the 60-Second Sweat has you covered. It is important to understand how essential it is to build an adequate level of fitness and then maintain it as we age. After the age of 30, if we don't do something to prevent it, we start to lose lean muscle every year. This makes it harder to maintain a healthy weight and makes us more prone to injury. Ultimately, it also puts us at greater risk for cancer, type 2 diabetes, heart disease, and all sorts of other nasty health problems.

Furthermore, maintaining fitness is critical to our ability to move well and without undue pain. Again, you need to have mobility, stability and strength, and flexibility in the areas which lack it. This means you need a program that addresses all of these components, which is exactly what the 60-Second Sweat does.

Bottom line: The days of inefficient, archaic, time-consuming, unsafe, and impractical fitness programs and workouts are over. Don't waste your valuable time and energy committing to an unrealistic regimen that will leave you bored, frustrated, (likely) hurt, and, in the end, stagnant, with absolutely zero change in your level of fitness, conditioning, or capacity to exercise more.

Instead, if you want to be able to continue to hit the slopes, play in your company softball tournament, feel confident in your swimsuit—or just keep up with your kids and get up off the floor without a challenge—then you need the 60-Second Sweat.

THE 60-SECOND PROMISE

Can elite fitness and the body of your dreams be built in one minute? No. I am not a huckster or snake oil salesman. I am an ethical fitness professional who understands the mind-set and expectations of the typical adult looking to get and stay in shape.

We all have a little ADD (attention deficit disorder), and, in my experience, this is especially the case when it comes to exercise. It is hard to keep anyone's attention. If you are like me, you have e-mails coming in, the phone ringing, texts and news feeds buzzing, the television on, and a subscription music service playing . . . all at the same time. If you want me to exercise—or do anything else, for that matter—it damn well better be varied, interesting, and effective! I don't want to be doing anything for too long or wasting my time in a world of competing demands for my attention. This is the society we live in: Everyone's looking for instant gratification, variety, what's shiny and new.

This is what the 60-Second Sweat is all about: keeping your attention and providing plenty of variety . . . but in a perfectly structured and progressive format. The best way I can describe it is "structured chaos." There are plenty of fitness programs out there that promise infinite variety.

That's all fine and good. However, most of these programs lack structure, comprehensiveness, and progression . . . rhyme and reason, if you will. You may have heard of the term periodization. Periodization is nothing more than the systematic variation of training variables over time (sets, repetitions, training volume, exercise progressions, etc.) The 60-Second Sweat uses periodization to help you keep progressing from a beginner, to an intermediate, to an advanced level of fitness.

The 60-Second Sweat is structured as a 9-week program made up of 3 separate 3-week phases. Each phase is made up of 2 to 3 different workouts, each in turn composed of several circuits of individual exercises.

During the 60-Second Sweat workouts, you will never be performing the same exercise or activity for more than 1 minute. There will be plenty of variety and, most importantly . . . it will be fun! And, unlike most other programs, every exercise, set, rep—every minute—will count for and toward something: developing the best and fittest you!

It would be easy for me to present a bunch of intense, cool-looking exercises that motivate you . . . until they don't. Eventually, you need to see results or you will go on to something else. The 60-Second Sweat program keeps your immediate attention, but, more important, the results you'll see—and the progressive and logical format—will keep you coming back time and time again to keep you invested over the long haul.

Get ready to experience the 60-Second Sweat difference! Let's delve into the principles that make the 60-Second Sweat so effective, and that will allow you to unlock your fitness potential . . . 1 minute at a time!

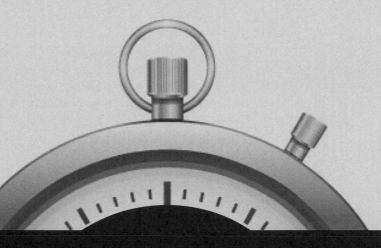

PART I

BEFORE YOU SWEAT

60-Second
Principles

As I mentioned in the introduction, there are thousands of appealing workouts on the fitness landscape. What separates the 60-Second Sweat from the rest of the pack is a cohesive set of principles, based on the real-world application of the most up-to-date exercise science, and modern strength and conditioning methods. Any program can look great on paper. However, unless it is usable over the long haul and produces results, it's just short-term "fluff" that, typically, will be abandoned and discarded by the end user—you.

The 60-Second Sweat is a program, not just a workout. It is not a short-term fix, but, rather, a road map to the fittest, most confident you. While the 60-Second Sweat workouts will certainly challenge you and leave you dripping in sweat, that's not the end goal. The purpose of the programs in this book is for you to attain phenomenal and sustainable strength, stability, mobility, flexibility, and cardiovascular fitness . . . safely and realistically . . . 1 minute at a time. Remember, whether your goal is to lose weight, feel and move better, improve your general fitness—or all three—the 60-Second Sweat has you covered.

I have taken great care in developing a realistic, safe, and effective program based on the following principles:

HIGH-INTENSITY INTERVAL TRAINING (HIIT)

High-Intensity Interval Training (HIIT) is the foundation upon which the 60-Second Sweat is built. HIIT, in very simple terms, is alternating bouts of intense exercise with less intense "rest" periods. For example, you might run as fast as you possibly can for the entire length of a football field and then walk around the end zone for 30 to 60 seconds before repeating again.

Why does this work? Exercise is like lighting a fire to your metabolism. When you are active, your metabolic flame and your caloric expenditure increases to varying degrees. With traditional, low- to moderate-intensity exercise—like walking on a treadmill or using an elliptical trainer for 30 minutes at a steady pace—you light the flame and it slowly increases to a gradual burn. When you end the workout, the flame dies down quickly and abruptly . . . kind of like dumping water on it.

On the contrary, with HIIT, the high-intensity exercise creates a huge metabolic disturbance and the flame heats up rapidly. Each interval is like squirting lighter fluid on the fire. What's more, after a HIIT workout, the flame gradually burns down and simmers for a long time. Have you ever lit a fire, let it burn all night, and found that the coals were still hot and glowing in the morning? That's HIIT, and that's the effect it has on your metabolism: It's intense, and you continue burning calories even when the workout is complete. This is called excess post-exercise oxygen consumption, or EPOC: Following an exercise session, oxygen consumption (and thus caloric expenditure) remains elevated as the working muscle cells restore physiological and metabolic factors in the cell to pre-exercise levels. This is what traditional cardio can't accomplish: A review article published in the *Journal of Sports Sciences* notes that exercise-intensity studies indicate higher EPOC values with HIIT training as compared with low- to moderate-intensity steady-paced cardiovascular training.[1] And it doesn't take long for these benefits to kick in. A team from the University of Guelph in Canada showed that fat oxidation, or fat burning, was significantly higher after 6 weeks of interval training.[2] Another study out of the University of Guelph showed a similar shift in as little as 2 weeks.[3]

HIIT also turns out to be better at developing cardiovascular fitness, or conditioning, than traditional cardio training. Cardiovascular function is often measured by maximal oxygen consumption, commonly called maximal aerobic capacity or VO_2max (maximal volume of oxygen). The uppermost ability of the body to consume, distribute, and utilize oxygen for energy production, VO_2max is a good predictor of exercise performance. In what is the most comprehensive (and recent) study comparing HIIT and traditional, longer-duration cardio, Jenna Gillen found that 12 weeks of sprint training (3 sessions per week for a total of 10 minutes per session) on a stationary cycle, consisting of only 3 20-second all-out sprints separated by 2-minute recovery periods, led to the exact same improvements (20 percent) in aerobic fitness and insulin resistance as 3 45-minute continuous sessions at a moderate intensity.[4] Think about that: The HIIT group exercised for only 6 hours—as compared to 27 hours in the traditional cardio group—and got the same results!

A French study measured VO_2max responses among two groups of men and women; one group participated in an 8-week HIIT program; the other, in a traditional steady-paced cardiovascular training program.[5] The HIIT group saw higher VO_2max increases (15 percent) than the group doing traditional steady-paced cardiovascular training (9 percent). Improving cardiovascular function and increasing VO_2max are major goals of patients who suffer from heart disease. For this reason, some cardiac rehabilitation centers are beginning to include interval-training sessions with heart disease patients. Results show improvements similar to traditional low-intensity cardio, but in a shorter time and with fewer sessions.[6]

The take-home message? When compared with traditional low- to moderate-intensity continuous cardio, HIIT will allow you to:

- Burn fat faster.

- Burn more calories after your workout is over.

- Develop the same or better cardiovascular conditioning in a fraction of the time.

The workouts in each phase of the 60-Second Sweat program will always incorporate HIIT: You will work really hard for less than a minute—the 60-second promise—and then you'll recover just long enough for you to do it again. This format will develop your cardiovascular fitness, which in turn can lower your blood pressure and cholesterol levels, protect against heart disease and diabetes, increase bone density, improve sleep quality, and even help you live longer.

METABOLIC RESISTANCE TRAINING (MRT)

Metabolic Resistance Training (MRT) is nothing more than loaded HIIT, or, put another way, HIIT with resistance. HIIT is traditionally performed using cardiovascular activities: running/ sprinting, cycling, stair stepping, rowing, using elliptical trainers, etc. But this neglects muscular fitness and the maintenance of lean body mass.

Remember what I stated in the introduction: After age 30, if we don't do something to prevent it, we will gradually lose muscle mass each year we age. This is a big problem. Your muscles, via your tendons, pull on your bones to move you. If you lose strength and muscle mass as you age, you cannot produce as much force, which means it will become harder and harder to move, much less live an active life and enjoy activities. Ever see an elderly person shuffle? Or someone unable to get up off the floor? This is due to a lack of muscular fitness and overall stability.

To prevent muscle loss, you need strength training (also sometimes called weight or resistance training). Strength training also increases your resting metabolic rate (the number of calories you burn at rest), improves insulin sensitivity, helps prevent type 2 diabetes, lowers blood pressure and cholesterol levels, increases bone mineral density, decreases lower back pain, and maintains and improves strength (obviously!). And, of course, it helps you look toned and trim.

With MRT, you stay true to the fundamental principles of HIIT—alternating brief bouts of hard work with periods of recovery—but you add in resistance with strength-training exercises. The synergy of MRT and HIIT develops both cardiovascular AND muscular fitness in a single, efficient, no-nonsense workout.

There is a big misconception out there that strength training cannot build cardiovascular fitness. It certainly can if it is programmed correctly. *Anything* that increases your heart rate and respiratory rate can improve your cardiovascular fitness. While strength training is not aerobic (meaning it does not rely on your aerobic energy system, which uses oxygen), it is cardiovascular. Do 20 loaded squats with a challenging weight and tell me you are not breathing heavier and your heart rate isn't up!

Research proves that strength-training exercises can boost cardiovascular fitness. In a 2010 study, after completing a treadmill test to determine VO_2max, 10 college-aged men did as many

2-handed kettlebell swings as they could in 12 minutes, using a 16-kilogram kettlebell (about 35 pounds). This is a loaded exercise, a perfect example of Metabolic Resistance Training. The average percentage of VO_2 (65.3 percent) seen in this study was within the training range (60 percent to 85 percent) recommended to improve cardiorespiratory endurance, so the authors concluded that this protocol "provided a metabolic challenge of sufficient intensity to increase VO_2max."[7]

Unless you are a current or an aspiring endurance athlete, you don't need to devote much time toward low-intensity (below 70 percent of your maximum heart rate), prolonged (exceeding 20 minutes) aerobic training. If your only goals are to feel better, move better, improve the tone of your entire or specific areas of your body, and look better naked . . . you can develop total fitness—cardiovascular and muscular—in a fraction of the time using MRT and HIIT.

MULTIPLE-JOINT EXERCISES

In order to get the most out of Metabolic Resistance Training and High-Intensity Interval Training, exercise selection is everything. Strength-training exercises can either be single-joint or multiple-joint. An example of a single-joint exercise would be a biceps curl, which recruits and works only one primary muscle (in this case, the biceps) across one joint (in this the case, the elbow). On the other hand, a multiple-joint exercise works several muscles simultaneously across many joints. Think about performing a weighted squat where you are recruiting muscles that cross your hips, knees, and ankles; you are working the front of your thighs, the back of your thighs, your rear end, the muscles of your core, etc.

The metabolic demand of multiple-joint exercises is much higher than that of single-joint exercises, meaning that you'll be burning more calories and challenging your cardiovascular system to a greater degree. The more muscle mass you can stimulate at one time, the better. When you are seeking to develop both strength and conditioning in the same workout, multiple-joint exercises are the way to go, and they make up the vast majority of the 60-Second Sweat programs. Again, we are looking for time efficiency, comprehensiveness, and return on investment: I will not be wasting much time having you isolate individual muscles, which lowers the overall intensity of any given workout. Single-joint exercises serve a purpose, but the 60-Second Sweat is not targeted toward bodybuilders or those recovering from an injury. The goal of the 60-Second Sweat is to develop functional, all-around fitness and health in a time-efficient package that fits the typical individual's busy life.

NON-COMPETING EXERCISES

Generally speaking, the exercises in the 60-Second Sweat workouts are performed in a non-competing fashion. In other words, an upper-body exercise will be followed by a lower-body exercise, which will then be followed by an exercise that targets the core and abdominals. In my 18 years of experience, I have found this is an ideal format for the general or beginning exerciser, as it is quite efficient. There is no need to perform a set of an exercise, rest, then perform another

⏱ 60 SECOND SUCCESS STORY

"I have always been a fitness enthusiast. Before I met Patrick, I had run 15 marathons and competed in triathlons on a weekly basis. But like many cardio junkies, I couldn't do a pull-up. I started working with Patrick after our third child was born and I couldn't carry the car seat without pulling my back out. After working with him for two years, I can say that I am in the best shape of my life. I am glad that I sought

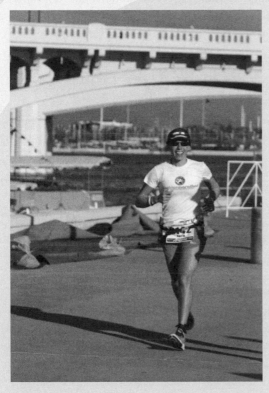

out Patrick's help, and because of him I have been able to take my fitness to the next level—squatting over 120 pounds, doing multiple pull-ups, and pressing 35-pound dumbbells over my head—which I never would have achieved on my own. His passion for fitness, knowledge of exercise science, and creativity makes him the very best trainer I have ever met. What's more? It is a true testament to his great work that I was able to carry my fourth pregnancy, with twins, to term without any pain or discomfort . . . and he had me back in pre-pregnancy condition less than 8 weeks after my delivery, which amazed me, my friends, and my family alike. Having 5 young children, 2 of them newborns, can be overwhelming, but Patrick's fitness 'recipe' has allowed me to take on each day with vigor and keep up without missing a beat. His workouts are perfect in that they are challenging and can be done in under 45 minutes but don't leave you completely depleted and unable to 'do' the rest of your hectic life."

—Katie O'Brien, 33, Cincinnati, OH

set of the same exercise. You'll actually get a greater bang for your buck (a more time-efficient workout in which you can perform a larger workout volume in the same amount of time) and better recovery between sets of the same exercise by pairing up one exercise with a second (and sometimes a third) that works a different or an opposing area of the body.

Far too many programs call for several exercises in a row targeting the same muscle groups. Unless you are advanced (having been consistently training for 3 or more days per week for 3 or more years), this will shorten your overall workout. All too often, I've seen people make it 10 to 15 minutes into a workout and then have to bow out quickly because they can hardly walk, cannot lift their arms, can't close their hands, or are nauseated. By performing non-competing exercises that work different areas of the body, the overall volume and intensity of the workout does not suffer. You can make it through the entire workout, but you also give specific muscle groups time to recover adequately while you work with different muscles.

COMPREHENSIVENESS & STRUCTURE

As a veteran fitness professional, I cannot tell you the number of times I've read workouts published in books and magazines and said to myself, "This author has clearly never trained anyone in the real world." Good programs and workouts need to flow. They need to be practical (not requiring specialized equipment), not too hard (or too easy) for the typical exerciser to perform, comprehensive (addressing all major muscle groups and all components of fitness), and safe (minimizing the risk of injury and not exacerbating any current orthopedic issue).

When I write training programs, I take everything into consideration . . . from exercise selection, to exercise pairings, to rest periods, and so on. I think about how the typical person will go through a workout, the equipment most people will have access to, and common orthopedic issues people may have, and I go by my experience. I know what people do and don't like, what they can and can't tolerate, and so on. Over 18 years, I've developed a real feel for this.

The 60-Second Sweat is comprehensive and structured to work all of your muscles. An equal amount of work is given to the upper body, lower body, and core musculature. Similarly, it is balanced between the front and back of the body. Too many modern fitness programs focus on the "mirror muscles": chest, front shoulders, front abs, and front arms. But the typical adult desk jockey needs to strengthen and activate the back of the body. Many of us sit at desks all day in a rounded posture. This leads to tight chest muscles, hunched shoulders, weak upper backs, aching lower backs, sore hips, and weak rear ends.

In the 60-Second Sweat, upper body exercises alternate between pushing (which works the chest, front shoulders, and back of the arms) and pulling (which works the back muscles, rear shoulders, and front of the arms). Lower-body exercises target either the front of thighs (quads) or the back (the hamstrings, lower back, and rear end). Core exercises rotate to target different areas (the front abdominals, lower abdominals, side abdominals, rear end, and lower back) or functions (flexing, extending, rotating, bending) of the core.

In addition to the strength-training portion of the program, I've also included time-efficient yet complete and thorough warm-up routines to prepare the body for the intense nature of Metabolic Resistance Training and High-Intensity Interval Training. You wouldn't start your car on a cold winter's morning and immediately floor the gas pedal. Your body is no different: You can't take it from 0 to 100 mph without a little warm-up. The warm-up protocols include both dynamic drills that mobilize specific areas of the body and traditional static stretching for commonly tight areas.

You may notice there is not a great deal of static stretching (longer duration holds of 20 to 60 seconds) in the 60-Second Sweat. You may be thinking, "Where is the stretching? Isn't that really beneficial to overall fitness?" Well, the more I've learned about static stretching, the less I've put it in the workouts I devise for my clients. Why? First of all, static stretching has a transient effect. You may stretch a muscle for a minute and feel good for a bit afterward, but it doesn't "stick," meaning that there are no long-term and long-lasting improvements in the range of motion for that joint.

Secondly, a lot of perceived tightness or inflexibility isn't due to actual short or stiff muscles. There is something called protective tension. If you move a specific joint through a certain range of motion and you're not strong enough to do so in a stable way, your body may sense it as a dangerous situation and your nervous system will literally shut things down so you don't hurt yourself. This has everything to do with a lack of strength and stability . . . not actual short muscles. If your body senses instability, it will shut movement down. Therefore, we should be focusing on getting stronger and more stable . . . not on trying to become Gumby.

Finally, some research is showing that if you stretch a muscle immediately prior to doing exercises intended to strengthen that muscle, you can actually diminish the strength of that muscle. Because stretching relaxes the muscle and its connective tendons, it will not fire with as much force when you are working it.[8] So you may find you actually need to use lighter weights or can't perform as many reps with a certain weight, so you get less benefit out of that workout.

And immediately after a workout, the muscles are too pumped up with blood to get a decent stretch. But I'm not throwing the baby out with the bathwater here or completely demonizing static stretching. There is some of it in your warm-up, as some areas are actually chronically short. However, static stretching makes up a very small component of this program. Your valuable time is better allocated elsewhere.

METABOLIC BLAST CIRCUITS

The final piece of the 60-Second Sweat workouts is what I've termed Metabolic Blast circuits. As I've mentioned, MRT and HIIT will develop total fitness—both strength and conditioning. The Metabolic Blast circuits are just the "icing on the cake"—a "finisher," if you will. The activities included in these circuits are more cardiovascular-oriented with a focus on power (the ability to produce force rapidly) and power endurance (the ability to continually produce force rapidly): low-level jumping, sprinting, changing directions, etc.

Most people know that we tend to lose strength—the ability to produce muscular force—as we age. However, few people realize that we also lose power—the ability to produce force and display strength rapidly. Many people want to continue participating in (or resume) recreational activities and sports they love. Many of these activities—driving a golf ball, playing basketball, getting down a black diamond ski slope, cutting and rotating on the tennis court—require explosive movements, during which you are rapidly changing directions or need to quickly accelerate or decelerate. These are skills you need to train for. The Metabolic Blast circuits address this by incorporating explosive movements in a safe manner.

PROGRESSION

Progression is what separates mere exercise from actual training. Exercise—what most people do when they go to the gym—is basically mindless mechanical work. Yes, it is activity—never a bad thing—but it is not structured, quantified, or progressive. In order to get fit, *you have to ask more of your body!* Period. If you do the "same ol' same ol'" and never ask more of yourself, there will be a point of diminishing returns as your body adapts.

The programs and workouts contained in this book systematically progress from a beginner stage (Break a Sweat) to an advanced stage (Dripping Sweat) over 9 weeks. You will be asked to do more, gradually and safely, over time. This may come in the form of more overall workout volume (more sets and reps), more difficult exercise progressions (going from a basic push-up from the floor to a push-up where you elevate your feet, for instance), shorter rest periods between exercises, or some combination of these. Rest assured, though, that it won't mean that it takes a lot more time!

A great level of fitness doesn't just happen; it's earned. I have formatted the workouts and programs in the 60-Second Sweat to ensure that you make progress and get consistently fitter over time, without being overwhelmed. If you try to progress too rapidly, you may end up too sore, injured, or loathing the experience so much that you quit. I think you'll find the progressive nature of 60-Second Sweat is very realistic and doable, leaving you motivated to come back for more each and every week.

TIME-EFFICIENT

As the name implies, the 60-Second Sweat is about all about efficiency. You just don't have hours and hours to spend in the gym. I get that and have crafted the workouts in this book accordingly.

In the beginner phase of the 60-Second Sweat, you'll be working out for around 30 minutes a day, 3 days a week. As you progress through the program, the duration may approach 40 minutes, 4 days a week, but absolutely no longer . . . and as you progress through the programs, you'll likely find it will take less time as your fitness rapidly improves.

And, in accordance with the 60-Second promise, all exercises within each workout will take 1 minute or less.

⏱ 60 SECOND SUCCESS STORY

"My commitment to a physically active lifestyle for a lifetime is as nonnegotiable today at age 67 as it was when I was a newly minted U.S. Army officer shipping off to Panama. Physical conditioning has contributed enormously to my maintaining a competitive edge in life—both personally and professionally. For over a decade, I've relied on Patrick Striet to keep my muscular strength, endurance, and flexibili-

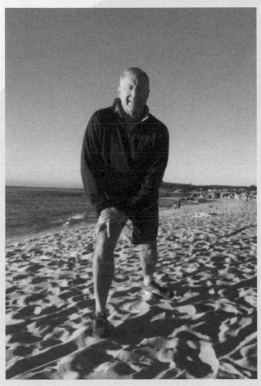

ty at the highest possible level. At 67, I'm able to bench-press 200 pounds and leg press over 300 pounds, and I can still row 500 meters in under 2 minutes . . . none of which would have been possible without Patrick's programming expertise.

"For the longest time, I thought there was no 'quick fix' to phenomenal fitness. What Patrick has taught me over the years is that, if your fitness program has structure, is based on sound principles, and is carried out consistently—in my case, just 2 workouts per week—quality will always trump quantity, and you can achieve great results with a very moderate time investment . . . and the programs in the 60-Second Sweat reflect that."

—Nelson Lees, 67, Cincinnati, OH

60-Second
Essentials

Now that you understand the foundational principles of this program, let's delve into the general workout guidelines and other information you need to know before you start the program. You might be tempted to skip straight to Part II to start sweating, but I definitely urge you to read through this chapter carefully before you do. It might seem a little boring, but here you'll find all the info you'll need to get the most out of the 60-Second Sweat.

WARM-UP

The warm-up portion of the 60-Second Sweat workouts is meant to prime your body for the harder work to come during the HIIT, MRT, and Metabolic Blast portions of the workouts. Both dynamic, movement-based drills and traditional static flexibility drills will be included in the warm-ups in order to mobilize certain areas (improving how joints move) and release typically tight muscles groups in other areas.

Do not skip or skimp on the warm-up! You cannot ask your body to go from 0 to 100 mph without prepping and preparing it. If you were parked in the driveway and it snowed 5 inches overnight, would you get in the car, start it up, and immediately hit the gas to back out? Or would you clean off the snow, start the car, and let it defrost and warm up? Hopefully the latter and not the former. Your body is the same way. Skipping a warm-up is hazardous, will more than likely lead to an injury, and will decrease performance during the main workout. Move through the warm-ups swiftly and deliberately, but give them their due attention. None of the warm-ups should take more than 5 minutes. Follow the specific instructions for each workout and program *exactly.*

⏱ 60 SECOND SUCCESS STORY

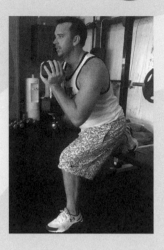

"By using Patrick's methods, I dropped 60 pounds and 15 percent body fat in 8 months! I never imagined when I started my journey under Patrick's guidance that I could achieve these types of results in only 3 workouts per week! Beyond the changes to my body, it has truly transformed my entire life: My energy levels and productivity are as high as they've ever been, and I'm a better husband, father, and business owner . . . and I actually LOOK FORWARD to working out for the first time in my life!"

—**Larry McGraw,** 36, Hebron, KY

FREQUENCY

I designed the 60-Second Sweat to be practical and fit your busy lifestyle. This is a real-world program for real-world people who can't go to the gym 5 days a week. In the Beginner and Intermediate phases of the program, you will train 3 days a week; in the Advanced phase, you'll work out 4 days a week.

Each phase is set up in a work day/rest day format, so you'll always have 24 hours to recover between workouts. You do not get stronger or more fit during your workouts: You simply provide the stimulus for that to happen. When you strength train, you are actually creating small tears in your muscle fibers. It's during your rest days, when your body repairs these tears, that your muscles get stronger. You have to allow your body to compensate after the stress of a hard workout and recover for you to see results, and this is the very goal of the recovery days.

So for those of you who become hypermotivated and may be tempted to do the 60-Second Sweat workouts more frequently, it is important to understand that more is not better. If you don't allow your muscles to recover adequately, you risk overtraining and injury, which would wipe out all your hard work. While it's perfectly fine to engage in other physical activities on scheduled rest days—such as leisurely walking, a hike in the woods, a round of golf, or other recreational sports—you don't want to do the 60-Second Sweat workouts 2 days in a row and you don't want to do them more than 3 to 4 times a week. You can get great results in just 3 to 4 days a week if you give the 60-Second Sweat workouts your all and follow the suggested guidelines.

And for those of you who find even a 3- to 4-day commitment daunting and unrealistic, I would first ask you to look at how you are spending your time. I often hear, "I don't have time to work out." But do you have time to binge watch TV, scour the Internet, post on social media, etc.? Everyone has the same amount of time in a given week. How you use that time is up to you. As far as I'm concerned, there is nothing better you could do with your time than investing in and prioritizing your health and fitness. At the very most, your commitment to the 60-Second Sweat will require 2.5 hours per week. Even for the busiest of us, I think this is realistic most of the time.

Another thing that can save you a great deal of time is setting up a simple home gym. The 60-Second Sweat requires only 4 pieces of equipment: dumbbells, a stability ball, an adjustable bench, and resistance bands. Purchasing these pieces of equipment—even used—is a very modest investment when you consider the return: better health and fitness. Setting up a home gym will spare you the commute to and from a gym and the crowds. For some, this is a very viable option.

That being said, I know everyone will still have some weeks when it's just not possible to fit in the 60-Second Sweat workouts as laid out in the weekly schedules. In those cases, see page 21 for guidelines on how to modify your schedule in the safest and most effective way possible.

TIME

Since you've picked up a book called 60-Second Sweat, my guess is that you are looking for a workout that doesn't take much time. Here's how I designed the program to deliver on that promise.

Strength-training exercises have a lifting (or concentric) phase and a lowering (or eccentric) phase. In the 60-Second Sweat, you should lift the weight quickly, in about 1 second. The lowering phase should be slower, taking 2 to 3 seconds. This means you need to control the weight as you lower it, rather than letting gravity do the work; this really works the muscles. You can lower approximately 40 percent more weight than you can lift, so in order to take advantage of that and optimally stress the muscles, you need to slow down the negative, or eccentric, phase of each repetition. If you cannot control the eccentric phase, you need to use a lighter weight. (It's always better to err on the side of going too light and being in control—then adding weight if you find that too easy—than going too heavy and risking injury.) You'll never do more than 15 repetitions (or reps) for each exercise (and in many cases, you'll do less), so assuming a 3- to 4-second rep, that's a 45- to 60-second set at most (a set, in fitness terminology, referring to one complete round of reps of any given exercise).

To keep up the intensity of the workouts, the rest period between sets and exercises never exceeds 30 seconds (and is often much less). Depending on the phase you're in, you'll do 6 to 12 exercises in a series of different circuits. In the Metabolic Blast portion of the workout, you'll alternate between 20 seconds of hard work and 10 seconds of rest on the prescribed activity. Depending on what phase you're in, you'll do this for 4 to 8 minutes.

Add in the 5-minute warm-up, and this adds up to a total workout of 30 minutes in the first 2 phases of the program and 40 minutes in the final phase. With that said, never sacrifice form, or the ability to complete an entire workout in order to complete it in less than 30 or 40 minutes. During the first few weeks, if you need to take a little more time between sets and exercises, it's perfectly fine. It's better to build your capacity to do more exercises—even if that means taking a little longer between sets and exercises—and complete the entire workout than to exhaust yourself quickly and be forced to do only a percentage of the workout. Don't worry . . . your conditioning will improve quickly, and you'll soon find you'll be able to adhere to the suggested rest intervals.

If you're really strapped for time and absolutely can't spend 30 minutes working out, see the guidelines on page 21 for the best way to adjust the program safely. All of the specific time guidelines as related to repetition speed, work, and rest intervals will be reinforced and reiterated in the program-specific guidelines.

INTENSITY

Intensity refers to how hard you are working. Intensity is both subjective (a general feeling of your effort level) and, when it comes to weight selection on the individual exercises, objective and quantified. Because the 60-Second Sweat incorporates High-Intensity Interval Training (HIIT) and Metabolic Resistance Training (MRT), it is, generally speaking, intense. The pace of the workouts, particularly the brief rest periods, is designed to challenge you, as is the nature of the multiple-joint exercises. They will have you breathing heavily, and if you are not, you need to increase the resistance you are using. The same can be said about the progressive nature of the overall program: increased volume (more sets and reps) and/or frequency (the number of days you are working out) and/or more difficult exercise progressions (for example, going from a push-up with your feet on the floor to a push-up where your feet are elevated).

However, you need to be smart. I certainly want you to follow the workouts as written, but this should never come at the expense of proper form, technique, and body alignment. If you feel your form is suffering—meaning you are using muscles not meant to be worked in a specific exercise or you are not feeling it in the targeted muscles—lower the resistance you are using or rest just a bit longer in between sets and exercises. As you'll see reiterated in the specific instructions for each phase of the 60-Second Sweat, I advise you to choose weights that allow for 1 or 2 more reps than what is prescribed. For instance, if I call for 3 sets of 10 repetitions of biceps curls, at the end of each set, you should feel as though you could do 1 or 2 more biceps curls, for a total of 36 curls. If your arms are trembling so much after doing just 8 or 9 biceps curls that you feel like you couldn't possibly do another, then you're using weights that are too heavy.

Going too heavy and altering your form is a no-no, but, on the flip side, going too light and not challenging yourself is just as bad. If an exercise calls for 12 reps, choosing a weight with which you can easily perform 20 or 30 reps will do absolutely nothing in terms of improving your muscular fitness. There needs to be a happy medium here: Choose a weight that allows you maintain your form and body alignment and allows you to feel the stress in the target muscles, but make sure you are challenging yourself . . . remember, only 1 or 2 reps left in reserve at the end of a set. This is a trial and error process. Don't worry if it takes a workout or two to find the sweet spot. What's likely to happen is that, after the first set of an exercise, you'll have a pretty good idea about whether you should increase or decrease the weight for the remaining sets.

Remember, the 60-Second Sweat is meant to develop all-around fitness: strength, conditioning, flexibility, and the ability to move well without pain. We are not trying to maximize absolute strength or muscle growth, nor do we want to emphasize any one component of fitness over another. Yes, there is a minimum threshold you to need to reach—1 or 2 repetitions shy of muscular exhaustion—but you do not need to train "all out" to complete exhaustion. In fact, if you do, you're not likely to be able to maintain the correct form. This may take the stress off the target muscles, rendering the exercise ineffective or, worse yet, leading to injury.

So how do you know when to increase the weight on an exercise? When you are able to complete all the suggested reps—in excellent form—for the number of sets called for in a particular phase, increase the weight slightly. In the case of dumbbell exercises, this means a 5-pound increment on a dumbbell and no more. You may find that by increasing the weight, you might not be able to complete all of the suggested reps on every set. That's perfectly fine. Just stick with this weight for the next workout(s), and try to add a rep or 2 to the sets in which you were unable to achieve the goal number on the prior workout or week. Remember, it's better to perform fewer perfect reps than a greater number of sloppy reps. What about band and body-weight exercises? Well, for band exercises, simply walking farther away from the anchor point—which develops more tension in the band—or using a stronger resistance band—will make the exercise harder. For body-weight exercises, you can simply perform more than the suggested number of repetitions or perform a more challenging variation of the exercise (for instance, once you've mastered the Single-Leg Glute Bridge, move on to the Single-Leg Hip Thrust).

EQUIPMENT

A downfall of many modern fitness programs is their reliance on specialized equipment. I've found many people are intimidated when they go to commercial gyms and fitness centers because they just don't know how to set up or use the equipment properly. While all those shiny chrome machines look nice, they are unnecessary.

The 60-Second Sweat requires a minimal amount of equipment found in every gym. You won't have to worry about figuring out the right seat settings, getting yourself lined up properly, or waiting on someone else to use the equipment. Sitting around waiting or spending time fiddling with equipment goes against the 60-Second promise and philosophy. You want an efficient, get-in-and-get-out workout, and with the 60-Second Sweat, you'll get just that.

While the 60-Second Sweat workouts are easily performed in a gym, they are also well suited for at-home exercisers. If this describes you, you'll find a list of the 4 basic pieces of equipment you'll need—as well as my recommendations on where to purchase them—below:

- **Dumbbells or set of adjustable dumbbells** (roguefitness.com or powerblock. com). For the vast majority of people utilizing the 60-Second Sweat, dumbbells ranging from 5 to 50 pounds (in 5-pound paired increments) will more than suffice and allow adequate progression. Generally speaking, most males will find weights between 25 and 50 pounds more than adequate for most of the dumbbell exercises in this program, while most women will find 15 to 40 pounds to be about right.

- **An exercise bench that adjusts from 0 to 90 degrees** (roguefitness.com). Do NOT attempt to substitute a table, chair, platform, exercise ball, etc., for a solid and well-designed adjustable bench as this will, first, open up the potential for injury, and second, make an exercise less effective and awkward.

- **A 55-cm stability/exercise ball** (performbetter.com)

- **All-purpose resistance bands with handles** (performbetter.com or elitefts.com)

In addition, a few exercises call for something on which to anchor your resistance band. For this purpose, what's most important is to find something solid and heavy that won't shift or slide as you pull on it. If you're in the gym, you can use the supports of most exercise machines. If you're at home, try a door frame, a bedpost, or a railing.

Finally, the following pieces of equipment are optional but may make your workouts easier and more comfortable:

- **An exercise mat** (performbetter.com)

- **An interval timer,** which will make the Metabolic Blast portion of your workouts go much more smoothly. I really like the Gym Boss (gymboss.com), but you can just as easily use an app on your smartphone or smart watch. Doing a quick search for "Tabata" or "Interval Timer" in the Apple and Android app stores will provide many options.

TRAINING LOG

I suggest that you keep a training log. Tracking your progress will help you stay motivated and allow you to see when you're ready to add weight or otherwise modify your workout to make it as effective as can be. The more precise you are in quantifying your workouts, the better your results will be. Don't attempt to guess what you did the prior workout or go from memory. Use a notebook or a computer spreadsheet and simply write down or log the following:

- In what order you did the exercises

- The name of the exercise

- The number of sets you performed for the exercise

- The rest period taken between each set of the exercise

- The amount of weight you used for each set of the exercise

- The number of repetitions completed on each set with a given weight

That's all you need. It does not need to be overcomplicated or fancy. Before you start a workout, take a quick look at your log and see what you achieved the prior workout . . . and then try to surpass it. It's that easy.

Here's a blank log sheet you can photocopy, or you can create your own:

ORDER	EXERCISE	SET	REST	WORKOUT 1				WORKOUT 2				WORKOUT 3				WORKOUT 4			
				WEIGHT		REPS		WEIGHT		REPS		WEIGHT		REPS		WEIGHT		REPS	
				GOAL	ACTUAL	GOAL	ACTUAL	GOAL	ACTUAL	GOAL	ACTUAL	GOAL	ACTUAL	GOAL	ACTUAL	GOAL	ACTUAL	GOAL	ACTUAL
		1																	
		2																	
		3																	
		1																	
		2																	
		3																	
		1																	
		2																	
		3																	
		1																	
		2																	
		3																	
		1																	
		2																	
		3																	
		1																	
		2																	
		3																	

PHASES

I designed this program to offer a safe and logical progression of workouts that work for the vast majority of general exercisers. Each phase builds on the one before it, like so:

1. Break a Sweat (Beginner Phase): This is a 3 day/week entry-level phase. The overall workout volume (sets and reps) is moderate, and the exercises are not too difficult to perform. This phase is suitable for those who exercise sporadically, have not exercised in years, or have never exercised before—but thanks to the intense nature of the MRT/HIIT workouts, it can still be challenging enough for those who already exercise regularly.

2. Hard Sweat (Intermediate Phase): This is a 3 day/week phase that is a step up from Break a Sweat. In this phase, you'll find a higher workout volume (more sets and reps), shorter rest periods between exercises, and more challenging exercises.

3. Dripping Sweat (Advanced Phase): This is the final 4 day/week phase, once again calling for a higher workout volume (more sets and reps), the most challenging exercises, extremely short rest periods, and an increased frequency of training. If you can complete these 3 weeks according the specific workout instructions, you will have achieved a terrific—and sustainable—level of fitness.

In all 3 phases, the workouts follow this basic structure:

1. Warm-Up: a brief (5-minute) protocol to mobilize, lengthen, turn things on, get you moving better, and increase core body temperature.

2. HIIT/MRT: a circuit of strength-training exercises utilizing the principles of High-Intensity Interval Training (HIIT) and Metabolic Resistance Training (MRT). This is the body of the workout and focuses on increasing both muscular fitness and cardiovascular conditioning.

3. Metabolic Blast Circuit: a 20 seconds on/10 seconds off circuit of body-weight cardiovascular exercises focusing on improving your cardio, power, and power endurance.

I chose to make each phase 3 weeks because I've found that it takes that long for my clients to really master the exercises, perfect their form, and work up to a challenging weight. But it's not so long that you get bored or start to do the exercises on autopilot, forgetting to check your form or increase your weight.

Within each phase, you can adjust the difficulty level by changing the amount of weight you're using or, in some cases, choosing between different variations of the same exercise (e.g., Push-Up, Bench Push-Up, or Kneeling Push-Up). So you can easily personalize the 60-Second Sweat to be challenging, but not too difficult, no matter what your current fitness level is.

That being said, I understand that the 3-week-per-phase progression may not work for everyone. Here are some guidelines to modify the phase progression if you need to:

⏱ 60 SECOND SUCCESS STORY

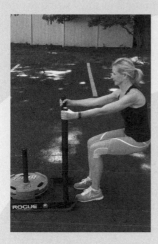

"Patrick Striet's fitness programs redefine your body. I am a successful executive who had to balance work and raising three children. I have worked with Patrick for over 8 years, and my body is in the best shape ever! What's more, during this time, he has come up with intelligent and effective strategies after my hip replacement and ACL reconstruction. I have excellent muscle tone and flexibility, and his program has helped to maintain my weight while also developing the ability to do perfect push-ups in my late 50s! Patrick's programs are structured so well that anyone can start, no matter your current physical activity or age, and you will see an improvement."

—**Donna Deye,** 57, Loveland, OH

- If you have been totally sedentary, are obese, or find that the workouts in the first phase are just too difficult: In Week 1 of the Break a Sweat phase, do the Warm-Up and just 1 or 2 circuits of the MRT/HIIT workout. You can also skip the Metabolic Blast portion of the workout if you find it too difficult. Then, over the next 2 weeks, gradually work up to the full suggested workouts.

- If you have consistently been working out (working out 2 or 3 days per week for at least 30 minutes) and find the Break a Sweat phase too easy: Skip the Break a Sweat phase entirely and move directly to the Hard Sweat phase. If you choose to do this, though, it doesn't mean you shorten the whole program by 3 weeks. Instead, stick with the Hard Sweat phase for an extra week or 2 before moving on to the Dripping Sweat phase. Similarly, do the Dripping Sweat an extra week or 2, for a total of 9 weeks.

OVERCOMING COMMON OBSTACLES

As a trainer, I've heard every reason under the sun why people can't exercise regularly. But here's the secret to meeting your goals: For every problem, there is a solution; you just need to figure it out. With the 60-Second Sweat, I've already given you a way around most of the common obstacles to working out. But if you find you are still having trouble with these all-too-familiar issues, here are some additional ideas for you:

- If you really can't get to the gym 3 or 4 days this week: Work out as many days as you can (even if it's only 1 or 2 days) and add in an additional circuit or 2 to those workouts (but never more than 2). Another option is to do 2 workouts in the same day, with several hours between workouts. For example, if you are slammed with work Monday through Thursday but you have some room to breathe on Friday, you could do your Day 1 workout Friday morning and your Day 3 workout Friday evening. You could then perform your Day 5 workouts Sunday morning (and, if you were in the Dripping Sweat phase, when you have 4 workouts per week, you could also do your Day 7 workout on Sunday evening). To make sure you give your muscles adequate time to recover, though, if you choose this option, never do more than 2 workouts in a day and make sure you leave at least 3 hours between workouts. And take a rest day after you do this.

- If you really can't spend 30 minutes in the gym at a time: Eliminate the Metabolic Blast circuit. The HIIT/MRT portion of the workout will adequately address both muscular fitness and cardiovascular fitness, so you will still get a great training effect even if you eliminate the Metabolic Blast. Alternatively, you can do half of a specific workout in the morning (for instance, the Warm-Up and 3 sets of Circuit 1) and the second half later in the day (3 sets of Circuit 2 and the Metabolic Blast). Or, and this is my least favorite option, simply cut one circuit out of the HIIT/MRT segment of the workout and/or cut the Metabolic Blast circuit in half (if an exercise calls for 5 rounds, do 2 or 3; if it calls for 3 rounds, do 1 or 2). Do NOT skip the warm-up: If you skip a warm-up and get hurt, you may be out of commission for a week or more, which means fewer gains in your level of fitness.

- If you are traveling: Because the 60-Second Sweat workouts are so time-efficient and use basic equipment, you'll find you can do them in most hotel gyms if that's an option for you. If not, you can at least bring your bands with you and substitute band or body-weight exercises that work the same body parts as the dumbbell exercises in your workout for the day.

- If you have a chronic health condition (such as heart disease or arthritis) or have previously suffered any injuries: As long as you are very careful with your form, don't get too aggressive trying to use heavy weights, and stick with the progression of the program as written, the 60-Second Sweat should be safe for you to perform. In fact, it should help you feel better in the long run and may even be able to help reverse some of your symptoms. That being said, I strongly advise you to consult your physician prior to beginning this or any exercise or nutrition program. A complete physical examination is highly recommended if you are sedentary, have high cholesterol, have high blood pressure, have

60 SECOND SUCCESS STORY

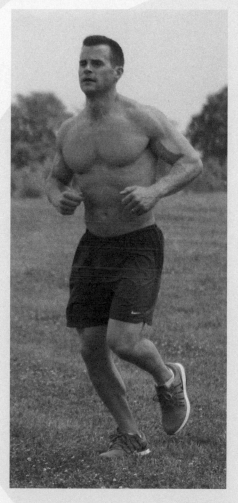

"I had always confused being busy with being productive, which had me in the gym 5 days a week focusing on the visible 'glamour' muscles. I thought that lifting for more than 15 years made me an expert, and though I looked fit, I was burned-out from doing the same back/bi, chest/tri, legs/shoulder exercises. After reading a *Men's Health* article about Patrick and Live Fit back in early 2014, I decided I needed a change and signed up for his distance-training regimen. I'm in medical sales, which means a lot of travel, stress, and long hours, so hiring a personal trainer that I would have to meet a few times a week was not an option for me. I discussed this with Patrick, and over the past two years, he has created customized, measurable, and efficient work-outs geared specifically toward me and my goals, making an impact that I didn't think was possible or attainable: squatting, bench pressing, and deadlifting over 300 pounds, doing 15 pull-ups, and taking my body fat to a level that turns heads on the beach.

"Patrick sends a different workout each month, and even though I'm only in the gym four to five hours per week at most, I continue to see gains in total-body strength and musculature. I'm 33 and have never been healthier or in better shape in my life. Patrick's distance training program has changed my 'check-the-box' attitude into one where I'm constantly challenging my mind and my body."

—Adam Yancey, 33, Union, KY

diabetes, are overweight, or are over 30 years old. You may also want to work with a personal trainer (and/or a registered dietitian if you choose to follow the 60-Second Sweat nutrition guidelines) in your first few weeks on the 60-Second Sweat program. It can really help to have a professional ensure that your form is correct and that you are using the appropriate weights.

60-Second
Nutrition

Obviously, I'm a big fan of fitness. In my 18 years as a trainer, I've seen firsthand the incredible benefits you can get just from doing workouts like the 60-Second Sweat. If you want to feel better, move without pain, and take your general fitness to a level you never imagined possible, the 60-Second Sweat program will deliver without you having to give your diet too much thought.

But if your goal is to lose weight, improve your body composition, and see all the shape and contour of the muscle you've built through your workouts? Well, that's a different story. If you want to significantly change the way you look, proper nutrition is absolutely essential. You cannot out-train a lousy diet.

Why? Think about how much time it takes you to eat a cheeseburger and french fries, a meal that probably exceeds 1,000 calories. Twenty minutes, maybe? Less, if you're really hungry? Now, how long would it take to burn that many calories? Well, jogging at 5 to 6 mph, for example, will burn about 10 calories a minute (that's dependent on your body weight, but this is a good average for most people). If we divide 1,000 by 10, that's 100 minutes of jogging to burn 1,000 calories. Twenty minutes to eat it and 100 minutes (over an hour and half) to burn it off. This is why exercise, by itself, stinks for weight loss. It's an efficiency issue.

So, while the 60-Second Sweat workouts will help build and shape all your muscles (in addition to many other benefits), you won't be able to see them if you are carrying too much body fat. If you want to get back into your skinny jeans or feel confident shirtless at the beach, you need to get your nutrition in order. The bottom line: Abs are made in the kitchen, and the best fat-loss exercise is 5 sets of stop eating so much crap! Without getting overly scientific or too in-depth, let's look at the key principles of 60-Second Nutrition.

SET AND ADHERE TO YOUR
CALORIE REQUIREMENTS

Rule number 1 of effective weight loss: Achieve a consistent caloric deficit, either by burning more calories, consuming fewer calories, or a combination of the two. As we've established, since burning more calories through exercise takes a lot of time and effort, eating less is the most efficient way to do this.

So how many calories should you be eating? Based on the scientific literature and my 18 years of practical experience designing nutrition programs for clients, consuming 10 to 12 calories per pound of your current body weight is safe and effective, and will put you in a slight calorie deficit. My advice is to start at the high end of the range (12 calories per pound) and see if you are dropping pounds, inches, and body fat. It's always better to see how much—not how little—you can eat and still lose fat. And although you may not want to hear it, losing weight slowly is the best route. If you drop your calories too low and lose too much weight too fast, you will likely be losing a lot of lean, metabolically active muscle tissue along with any weight and fat. Not good. Furthermore, the chance that your body will fight back, meaning you feel deprived and ravenous and go on a binge, is more likely.

Say, for example, that you weigh 150 pounds. Multiply that by 12, and you get 1,800 calories to eat per day (plus or minus 150 calories). Stick with that calorie level for 2 weeks. Evaluate your results. Keep in mind that the scale doesn't tell the entire story. Your weight can shift up and down drastically based on how much water you are holding, time of the month (for women), carbohydrate intake, water intake, "toilet status," and so on. So try to replicate the same conditions each week when you weigh yourself. For example, maybe it's every Wednesday right after waking up and going to the bathroom. In addition to weighing yourself, I suggest that you take hip, waist, thigh, upper-arm, and calf measurements. If you have access to someone competent in taking body-composition (skin-fold calipers) measurements, that's a great addition as well. Another great tool? The mirror. How do you look? Do you have more defined muscles? Less dimpling? Does your waist look smaller? Have a friend or spouse take biweekly photos from the front, back, and side, and compare the photos every 2 weeks. Visuals go a long way and—pun intended—give a much better picture of what's going on.

After 2 weeks, if you haven't seen any changes, go just a bit lower in calories—say, to 11 calories per pound, or 1,650 calories daily. Fat loss and weight loss is never a linear process and never works out exactly by the numbers. I've seen many, many people not drop any pounds, fat or inches for 2 weeks at a certain calorie level, and then, "poof," it starts coming off! There are no absolutes in the world of nutrition, just guidelines.

One other thing to keep in mind: As you lose body weight and fat, your calorie requirements (unfortunately) decrease. So for instance, if you dropped 5 pounds to 145 pounds, your calorie requirements fall from 1,800 calories to about 1,740 calories per day. Each time you drop 5 pounds or more, recalculate and adjust your calorie level until you reach your goal weight. Once you reach your goal weight, stay at your latest calorie level.

EAT ENOUGH PROTEIN

Protein is the cornerstone of 60-Second Nutrition. Protein helps build and repair muscle and supports hard strength training. It helps keep you full and fends off cravings. Perhaps most importantly, it is a "metabolically expensive" macronutrient. Let me explain. There is a component of metabolism called the Thermic Effect of Feeding (TEF). TEF is the amount of energy it takes to digest, absorb, and process the food we eat, and the 3 macronutrients (protein, carbohydrate, and fat) have different TEF values:

- **TEF value of protein:** 20 to 35 percent of calories burned through processing

- **TEF value of carbohydrate:** 5 to 15 percent of calories burned through processing

- **TEF value of fat:** 0 to 5 percent of calories burned through processing

What does this mean? Let's say you eat 100 calories of pure protein (for instance, a chicken breast). Due to protein's TEF, your body absorbs only 65 to 80 of those 100 calories, because the rest were burned in processing. But when you eat 100 calories of carbohydrate (such as a slice of white bread), your body absorbs 85 to 95 of those calories. When you eat fat (think butter or lard)? You'll absorb nearly all of it.

I hope it's apparent that consuming more protein is an easy way to create the necessary caloric deficit without really trying. That being said, you don't want to eat all protein, all the time, as the other 2 macronutrients—carbohydrate and fat—greatly benefit your health, fitness, and performance as well.

So how much should you eat? A study published in 2011 in the Journal of Sports Sciences supports the generally agreed-upon rule that you should shoot for (but not exceed) 1 gram of protein per pound of body weight per day.[9] If, as in our example above, you weigh 150 pounds, you should shoot for about 150 grams (or about ⅓ of a pound) of protein daily. Protein contains 4 calories per gram, so 150 grams of protein will give you about 600 calories, or a third of your daily allotment of 1,800 calories. Here's an example of how you could meet that requirement in a day:

- **Breakfast:** 4 eggs (28 grams of protein)

- **Lunch:** 6 ounces chicken breast (30 grams of protein)

- **Midafternoon:** 2 scoops of protein powder in water (48 grams of protein)

- **Dinner:** 6 ounces eye of round steak (36 grams of protein)

If you have been trying to cut back on meat consumption or sticking to lean protein for health or any other reasons, you can certainly still do so, but for the purposes of this program, any protein source is fine.

DON'T DEMONIZE FATS AND CARBS

Okay, so I've had all these glowing things to say about protein, but what about the other 2 macro-nutrients, carbohydrate and fat? Both of these have been demonized at certain points in time. Remember the '90s? Fat was public enemy number 1. The fat-free craze planted its roots and grew like mad. An entire industry developed from the fear of dietary fat. What happened? People ignored their overall calorie consumption, and obesity rates soared. Eating fat doesn't make you fat—eating more calories than you expend does. Eating fat can strengthen your immune system and your bones; improve your brain function and your mood; and keep your skin, eyes, and re-productive system healthy. Plus it's satiating, so you will feel fuller longer.

In the 2000s, carbohydrates replaced fat as the culprit of obesity. Low- and no-carb diets became all the rage (and certain "gurus" made a lot of money). Everyone was sitting down to huge plates of bacon and eggs and devouring steak. What happened? Again, obesity rates increased. Let me reiterate: Eating carbohydrates does not make you fat—eating more calories (from any source) than you expend does.

Carbohydrates are your body's main source of fuel. When you take in food, your body breaks down its sugars and starches and absorbs them into your bloodstream. At this point, they become glucose (blood sugar). Your body needs glucose to have the energy to do everything from breathing to strength training. In addition, your brain needs glucose to function properly. If you don't take in enough carbohydrates, you can become weak, lethargic, irritable, and unable to focus on even simple tasks. Plus, carbohydrates are the source of fiber in your diet. Fiber adds bulk to your diet, helping you to feel full, and can help prevent digestive problems and heart disease. Don't even think about undertaking the 60-Second Sweat training program on a low-carb diet. You'll crash and burn. Carbs are your preferred source of energy for the high-intensity exercise you'll be doing on the 60-Second Sweat.

What is the right amount of fat and carbs? I am a proponent of a fairly even distribution of the 3 macronutrients. Remember that in our example, you are 150 pounds and eating 150 grams, or about 600 calories worth of protein. That leaves 1,200 calories to devote toward carbs and fat, or 600 calories each. Carbs, like protein, contain 4 calories per gram, so you should eat 150 grams of carbs. Fat contains 9 calories per gram, so your goal is 600 calories divided by 9, or 66 grams of fat. As with protein, meeting these requirements is rather easy:

- **Breakfast:** 40 grams of quick oats, a medium apple (52 grams of carb), and 2 table-spoons all-natural peanut butter (16 grams of fat)

- **Lunch:** 200 grams of white sticky rice (75 grams of carb) and ½ cup of shredded sharp cheddar cheese (18 grams of fat)

- **Dinner:** 1 small sweet potato (26 grams of carb) and 2 ounces of raw almonds (30 grams of fat)

Again, if you have been trying to eat whole grains instead of processed ones or aiming for more monounsaturated fats than saturated or trans fats, that's great. But for the purposes of this program, there's no need to get that detailed. Just plug your own numbers in, and you have yourself a great fat-loss nutrition plan! One thing to note: There is nothing wrong with increasing the percentage of carbohydrate, especially given the training you'll be doing. If you feel you want to up your carb intake to 40 to 50 percent of your diet—and correspondingly reduce the percentage of fat—go for it. In fact, if you feel your workouts are lagging, you feel lethargic, etc., that's exactly what you should do. Again, you will NOT get fat eating a greater percentage of carbs if you do not exceed your caloric requirements!

At this point, you may be asking yourself, "Is all this number crunching, tracking, and quantification really necessary? I mean, can't I just eat a little better and still shed a lot of fat?" I hear this a lot and my typical response is, "Do you want decent results or optimal results?" If you just want to shed a few pounds and a little fat, making what I like to call "qualitative changes" to your nutrition may be all you need to achieve your goal. If your current diet is horrendous, going from 3 sausage, egg, and cheese biscuits to egg whites and oatmeal—without doing all the math—is likely going to yield positive results—for a while anyway. However, if you have a great deal of fat to lose—or stall with a "trying to eat better" approach—you will at some point have to dial things in, track, quantify, and weigh your food.

DON'T GO FOR VARIETY

You have probably heard you should eat a varied diet and include many, many different foods. Well, after 18 years of working with clients looking to shed fat and look better naked, I can tell you too much dietary variety is a recipe for disaster. You will have enough number crunching going on, and constantly introducing new foods will make you want to scream. Keep it very simple. Pick 4 to 5 sources of protein, carbs, and fat, and get familiar with them. For example:

- **Protein:** skinless chicken breast, tilapia, lean top sirloin, protein powder

- **Carbs:** rice, sweet potatoes, old-fashioned plain oatmeal, fruit

- **Fat:** olive oil, full-fat cheddar cheese, avocado, raw nuts

What about vegetables? The nice thing about vegetables—besides the phenomenal vitamins, minerals, micronutrients, and fiber contained within them—is that they contain very, very few calories. All non-starchy carbs are fair game, and you should indulge as you'd like! So think spinach, romaine lettuce, spring mixes, kale, chard, bell peppers, asparagus, onions, etc. However, be very careful not to dump high-calorie dressings, oils, and sauces on these, as you could easily find yourself overshooting your caloric needs.

PUTTING IT ALL TOGETHER

If your head is spinning with all these numbers, relax! It may take a little while to get used to, but once you get the hang of it, 60-Second Nutrition should take no more time than the workouts. Here's an example of how you could put together an 1,800-calorie meal plan according to the 60-Second Nutrition principles.

If these meals don't appeal to you, no problem! This is just an example—feel free to customize your meal plan to suit your tastes and your specific requirements.

1,800-CALORIE MEAL PLAN

MEAL	FOOD EATEN	AMOUNT	UNIT	PROTEIN GRAMS	CARB GRAMS	FAT GRAMS	CALO-RIES
BREAKFAST	Eggs	2	whole	12	1	10	142
	Egg whites	4	whites	14	0	0	56
	Quick-cooking oats	28	g	3.7	18.9	1.8	106.9
	Almond butter	28	g	6.1	5.3	15.8	187.3
	Steamed broccoli	1	cup	6	12	0	62
				41.8	37.2	27.6	554.2
LUNCH	Turkey breast	5	oz	32.5	0	2.5	152.5
	Bread, whole wheat	2	slices	10	40	2	218
	Raw cashews	28	g	5.1	8	12.3	163
	Raw bell peppers and baby spinach	1	cup	1	3.5	0	18
				48.6	51.5	16.8	551.5
DINNER	Grilled chicken breast	150	g	47.3	0	5.3	236.8
	Brown rice	140	g	3.2	32.2	1.3	153.4
	Liquid fish oil	2	tsp	0	0	10	90
	Sautéed asparagus	1	cup	4.5	7	0.5	50
				55	39.2	17.1	530.2
SNACK	Almond milk	1	cup	1	2	3	39
	Vanilla protein powder	1	scoop	25	5	4	156
	Banana	1	medium	1	27	0	112
				27	34	7	307
		Total:		172.4	161.9	68.5	1,942.9

PERCENT PROTEIN OF TOTAL CALORIES CONSUMED:		35.5
PERCENT CARBOHYDRATE OF TOTAL CALORIES CONSUMED:		30.7
PERCENT FAT OF TOTAL CALORIES CONSUMED:		33.7

TIPS & TOOLS OF THE TRADE

Failing to prepare is preparing to fail. Given the amount of number crunching I'm recommending, you want to make this process as easy and streamlined as possible. Here are my top recommendations:

1. Measure your food: When it comes to precision nutrition, a food scale is your best friend. You can find food scales at many retailers (Target and Bed Bath & Beyond, for example) or online (amazon.com). Most digital scales can be purchased for under $30. Make sure the scale weighs in both grams and ounces and can be reset to zero even if an item is on the scale.

2. Download a nutrition-tracking app: While this isn't absolutely necessary, an app can help you track your calorie and nutrient intake throughout the day. There are dozens of options in the app store. I like My Macros+ but there are plenty others. It comes down to personal preference. Perhaps download a few, play with them, and see what you like. A food-substitution app (I like Go Figure) is extremely helpful if you want to substitute one food for another (tilapia in place of your normal chicken, for example) and need to know what amount of the substituted food is the same number of calories.

3. Plan and prep your meals ahead of time: I cannot stress this enough. Once you've set your caloric requirements and figured out the amount of protein, carbs, and fat you need, take some time to make a meal plan. It's much easier to stick to your calorie and nutrition goals if you have mapped out your meals in the correct portions and prepped your food ahead of time. That means deciding what you'll eat for breakfast, lunch, and dinner for the week; getting to the grocery store to buy all the necessary ingredients; and cooking all or most of your meals for the next day or even for a few days. If you don't have the food in the house or don't have it prepared when you're hungry, you are much more likely to resort to takeout. This may seem like a no-brainer, but you'd be surprised at how many people I've coached over the years who have a real issue with getting to the store or prepping meals ahead of time.

4. Equip your kitchen: Prepping your meals ahead of time—and taking your meals "to go" if you need to—will be much easier if you have the right equipment. I strongly recommend that you invest in the following (many of which you probably already have in your house): a slow cooker (which allows you to easily cook meat in bulk overnight), measuring cups, plenty of plastic containers, shaker bottles, plastic utensils, a soft-sided cooler and ice packs (all of these make eating on the go and transporting your food a breeze).

5. Drink water: Keep yourself hydrated. My recommendation is half of your body weight in ounces. For example, if you weigh 150 pounds, shoot for 75 ounces daily. Things like flavored water drops (Mio and Crystal Light drops, for example) and fresh fruits, vegetables, or herbs (lemons, limes, mint, cucumbers, berries, etc.) are fine to put in your water. Outside of water, avoid calorie-containing drinks (soda, sports drinks, fruit juices, etc.): They are full of sugar and empty calories, which don't fill you up. Diet sodas are fine in moderation.

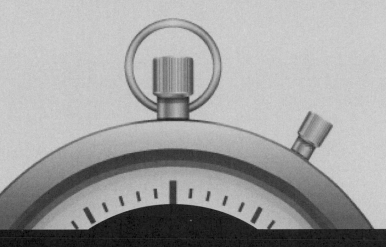

PART II

60 SECOND SWEAT PROGRAM

Break a Sweat
(Beginner Phase)

You can't walk before you can crawl. If you have not followed any formal type of exercise program in months or years, exercising only sporadically or not at all, this is where your journey begins. Break a Sweat is meant to establish a base level of fitness so that you can progress through the remaining phases of the 60-Second Sweat program safely and with confidence. Some of the exercises in these workouts may look or sound really tough, but trust me and try them. I've worked with many clients over the years who had never exercised before, had back or other issues, or were morbidly obese, and they were able to perform these exercises.

Follow the Break a Sweat phase for 3 weeks before progressing to the next phase, Hard Sweat. Remember that you can always make the exercises more challenging by adding more weight or adding a couple of additional repetitions to each set. But if you've done that and still find that after a week or two, you are ready for more, you can move to phase 2, Hard Sweat, a little early. Again, if you do this, just adjust the length of the other phases so that you follow the program for a total of 9 weeks. And, as noted in 60-Second Essentials, if you have been consistently following a structured exercise program (working out 2 or 3 days per week for at least 30 minutes), you may skip this phase entirely and instead start with phase 2, Hard Sweat, adjusting the length of the phases accordingly.

Be sure you have read all of the general workout guidelines and safety tips in 60-Second Essentials, as well as the Break a Sweat–specific guidelines that follow. Let's get to it!

WORKOUT GUIDELINES

Disclaimer: It is strongly advised that you consult your physician prior to beginning this or any other exercise or nutrition program. A complete physical examination is highly recommended if you are sedentary, have high cholesterol, have high blood pressure, have diabetes, are overweight, or are over 30 years old.

- Work out 3 days per week, alternating between workout A and workout B. So, in week 1, you'll perform the workouts in an A/B/A format, resting one day in between each workout. In week 2, you'll perform the workouts in a B/A/B format, etc. You'll continue in this format for the full 3 weeks.

- "20 on, 10 off" means you will work very hard for 20 seconds, followed by a period of rest for 10 seconds.

- Do not skip the warm-up routine outlined in this program!

- Don't train to failure/exhaustion. You should be able to do 1 more rep at the end of each set. If you can't, reduce the amount of weight you're using. Alternatively, if you find the weight to be far too easy for the suggested number of reps, increase the weight conservatively (by no more than 5 pounds at a time).

- If your time is limited, reduce the number of sets in the workout but do not, under any circumstances, skip the warm-up.

WEEKLY SCHEDULE	
Day 1	Workout A or B
Day 2	Recovery Day
Day 3	Workout A or B
Day 4	Recovery Day
Day 5	Workout A or B
Day 6	Recovery Day
Day 3	Recovery Day

WARM-UP

Perform the 6 exercises below in order, resting only as long as it takes to transition between exercises. Rest 30 to 60 seconds, then repeat the entire circuit.

	EXERCISE	REPS	REST
	Side-Lying Rotation (page 62)	6 reps/side	5 seconds rest/transition
	Glute Bridge (page 64)	10 reps	5 seconds rest/transition
	Quad/Hip Flexor Mobilization* (page 66)	6 reps/side	5 seconds rest/transition
	Cat/Camel Drill (page 70)	10 reps	5 seconds rest/transition
	Chest Stretch (page 74)	20 seconds/side	5 seconds rest/transition
	Lat Stretch (page 76)	20 seconds/side	5 seconds rest/transition

*If you need to hold on to something for balance, feel free to do so.

WORKOUT A

WORKOUT CIRCUIT #1

Repeat 3 times with a 20-second rest between exercises. Rest 1 minute between circuits.

EXERCISE		REPS	REST
	Stability Ball Leg Curl (page 170)	12 reps	20 seconds rest/transition
	3-Point Dumbbell Row (page 126)	10 reps/side	20 seconds rest/transition
	Plank (page 178)	30 seconds	

WORKOUT CIRCUIT #2

Repeat 3 times with a 20-second rest between exercises. Rest 1 minute between circuits.

EXERCISE		REPS	REST
	Dumbbell Goblet Squat (page 136)	12 reps	20 seconds rest/transition
	Push-Up, Bench Push-Up, or Kneeling Push-Up* (pages 82, 84, 86)	12 reps	20 seconds rest/transition
	Band Core Press (page 208)	5 reps/side (Hold in the extended position for 5 seconds on each rep.)	

*Your choice here depends on your fitness level. The first time you do this workout, experiment with all 3 variations over the 3 sets to determine which one is challenging yet doable.

METABOLIC BLAST CIRCUIT

EXERCISE	REPS	REST
Jumping Jacks (page 238)	20 on/10 off x 3 rounds	45 seconds rest
Mountain Climber (page 234)	20 on/10 off x 3 rounds	45 seconds rest
Full-Body Extension (page 224)	20 on/10 off x 3 rounds	

WORKOUT B

WORKOUT CIRCUIT #1

Repeat 3 times with a 20-second rest between exercises. Rest 1 minute between circuits.

EXERCISE	REPS	REST
Incline Dumbbell Chest Press (page 100)	12 reps	20 seconds rest/transition
Alternating Body Weight Reverse Lunge (page 156)	12 reps	20 seconds rest/transitionn
Stability Ball Crunch (page 198)	12 reps	

WORKOUT CIRCUIT #2

Repeat 3 times with a 20-second rest between exercises. Rest 1 minute between circuits.

EXERCISE	REPS	REST
Chest-Supported Dumbbell Row (page 124)	12 reps	20 seconds rest/transition
Hip Thrust (page 166)	15 reps	20 seconds rest/transition
Double-Arm Dumbbell Carry (page 190)	40 steps	

METABOLIC BLAST CIRCUIT

EXERCISE		REPS	REST
	Side-to-Side Shuffle (page 220)	20 on/10 off x 3 rounds (5 yards each direction)	45-second rest
	Body Weight Thruster (page 232)	20 on/10 off x 3 rounds	45-second rest
	Short Shuttle Run (page 222)	20 on/10 off x 3 rounds (5 yards each direction)	

Hard Sweat
(Intermediate Phase)

It's time to pick it up! Progressive overload—asking more of your body—is how fitness is built. Now that you've completed 3 weeks of Break a Sweat, it's time to push things further . . . and your body is ready for it. In this phase, we are going to increase the overall volume (adding more sets and reps) as well the difficulty of the exercises performed.

You should perform the Hard Sweat program for 3 weeks before progressing to the next phase, Dripping Sweat. Again, remember that you can make the exercises more challenging by adding weight. But if you've done that and after a week or two you still feel like the workouts are too easy, feel free to move to phase 3, Dripping Sweat. (Just adjust the length of the phases to make sure this stays a 9-week program.) Be sure you have read all of the general program guidelines and safety tips in 60-Second Essentials as well as the Hard Sweat–specific guidelines that follow. Onward and upward!

WORKOUT GUIDELINES

Disclaimer: It is strongly advised that you consult your physician prior to beginning this or any other exercise or nutrition program. A complete physical examination is highly recommended if you are sedentary, have high cholesterol, have high blood pressure, have diabetes, are overweight, or are over 30 years old.

- Work out 3 days per week, doing workouts A, B, and C in order through the week.

- "20 on, 10 off" means you will work very hard for 20 seconds, followed by a period of rest for 10 seconds.

- Do not skip the warm-up routine outlined in this program!

- Don't train to failure/exhaustion. You should be able to do 1 more rep at the end of each set. If you can't, reduce the amount of weight you are using. Alternatively, if you find the weight to be far too easy for the suggested number of reps, increase the weight conservatively (by no more than 5 pounds at a time).

- If your time is limited, reduce the number of sets in the workout but do not, under any circumstances, skip the warm-up.

WEEKLY SCHEDULE	
Day 1	Workout A
Day 2	Recovery Day
Day 3	Workout B
Day 4	Recovery Day
Day 5	Workout C
Day 6	Recovery Day
Day 7	Recovery Day

WARM-UP

Complete the 10 exercises below, resting only as long as it takes to transition between exercises.

EXERCISE	REPS	REST
Side-Lying Rotation (page 62)	6 reps/side	
Glute Bridge (page 64)	10 reps	
Quad/Hip Flexor Mobilization* (page 66)	6 reps/side	
Half-Kneeling Groin Mobilization (page 68)	6 reps/side	
Cat/Camel Drill (page 70)	10 reps	
Bird Dog (page 72)	6 reps/side	
Arm Circles (page 78)	10 reps each direction	
Arm Crosses (page 80)	10 reps	
Chest Stretch (page 74)	20 seconds/side	
Lat Stretch (page 76)	20 seconds/side	

*If you need to hold on to something for balance, feel free to do so.

WORKOUT A

WORKOUT CIRCUIT #1

Repeat 4 times with a 15-second rest between exercises. Rest 45 seconds between circuits.

EXERCISE	REPS	REST
Dumbbell Romanian Deadlift (page 172)	12 reps	15 seconds rest/transition
Alternating Band Row (page 120)	10 reps/side	15 seconds rest/transition
Stability Ball Rollout (page 202)	10 reps	

WORKOUT CIRCUIT #2

Repeat 3 times with a 15-second rest between exercises. Rest 45 seconds between circuits.

EXERCISE	REPS	REST
Dumbbell Front Squat (page 142)	12 reps	15 seconds rest/transition
Feet-Elevated Push-Up, Push-Up, or Bench Push-Up* (pages 82,86,88)	12 reps	15 seconds rest/transition
High-to-Low Band Chop (page 212)	10 reps/side	

*Your choice here depends on your fitness level. The first time you do this workout, experiment with all 3 variations over the 3 sets to determine which one is challenging yet doable.

WORKOUT CIRCUIT #3

Repeat 3 times with a 15-second rest between exercises. Rest 45 seconds between circuits.

	EXERCISE	REPS	REST
	Rear Foot-Elevated Split Squat (page 150)	8 reps/side	15 seconds rest/transition
	Single-Arm Dumbbell Push Press (page 110)	8 reps/side	15 seconds rest/transition
	Dying Bug (page 206)	5 reps/side (alternating)	

METABOLIC BLAST CIRCUIT

	EXERCISE	REPS	REST
	Band Swimmer (page 228)	20 on/10 off x 5 rounds	45 seconds rest
	Full-Body Band Extension (page 226)	20 on/10 off x 5 rounds	

WORKOUT B

WORKOUT CIRCUIT #1

Repeat 4 times with a 15-second rest between exercises. Rest 45 seconds between circuits.

	EXERCISE	REPS	REST
	Seated Dumbbell Shoulder Press (page 106)	12 reps	15 seconds rest/transition
	Alternating Goblet Reverse Lunge (page 158)	8 reps/side	15 seconds rest/transition
	Stability Ball Saw (page 204)	10 reps	

WORKOUT CIRCUIT #2

Repeat 3 times with a 15-second rest between exercises. Rest 45 seconds between circuits.

	EXERCISE	REPS	REST
	Bent-Over Band Lat Pulldown (page 132)	12 reps	15 seconds rest/transition
	Supported Body Weight Single-Leg Romanian Deadlift (page 174)	8 reps/side	15 seconds rest/transition
	Hollow Body Hold (hands placed across chest) (page 194)	20 seconds	

WORKOUT CIRCUIT #3

Repeat 3 times with a 15-second rest between exercises. Rest 45 seconds between circuits.

	EXERCISE	REPS	REST
	Dumbbell Crush Press (page 102)	12 reps	15 seconds rest/transition
	Jump Squat (page 144)	8 reps	15 seconds rest/transition
	Overhead Dumbbell Carry (page 192)	20 steps/side	

METABOLIC BLAST CIRCUIT

	EXERCISE	REPS	REST
	Short Shuttle Run (page 222)	20 on/10 off x 5 rounds (5 yards each direction)	45 seconds rest
	Cross-Body Mountain Climber (page 236)	20 on/10 off x 5 rounds	

WORKOUT C

WORKOUT CIRCUIT #1

Repeat 4 times with a 15-second rest between exercises. Rest 45 seconds between circuits.

EXERCISE	REPS	REST
Dumbbell Thruster (page 112)	12 reps	15 seconds rest/transition
Dumbbell Sumo Squat (page 140)	12 reps	15 seconds rest/transition
Plank Walk-Up (page 180)	6 reps/side	

WORKOUT CIRCUIT #2

Repeat 3 times with a 15-second rest between exercises. Rest 45 seconds between circuits.

EXERCISE	REPS	REST
Dumbbell Pullover (page 134)	12 reps	15 seconds rest/transition
Dumbbell Step-Up (page 154)	8 reps/side	15 seconds rest/transition
Low-to-High Band Chop (page 214)	10 reps/side	

WORKOUT CIRCUIT #3

Repeat 3 times with a 15-second rest between exercises. Rest 45 seconds between circuits.

EXERCISE	REPS	REST
T-Rotation Push-Up or T Rotation* (pages 94, 96)	6 reps/side	15 seconds rest/transition
Rear Foot-Elevated Isometric Split Squat (page 152)	15 seconds/side	15 seconds rest/transition
1 Back/1 Out Crunch (hands placed across chest) (page 200)	6 reps/side	

*Your choice here depends on your fitness level. The first time you do this workout, experiment with both variations over the 3 sets to determine which one is both challenging yet doable.

METABOLIC BLAST CIRCUIT

EXERCISE	REPS	REST
Body Weight Prisoner Squat (page 240)	20 on/10 off x 5 rounds	45 seconds rest
Run in Place (page 216)	20 on/10 off x 5 rounds	

Dripping Sweat
(Advanced Phase)

Congratulations! You've reached the last phase of the 60-Second Sweat program, Dripping Sweat. The ability to tackle Dripping Sweat indicates you've built a tremendous level of fitness over the past 6 weeks. The 3 weeks of Dripping Sweat will be your toughest challenge yet. In Dripping Sweat, we increase the frequency—to 4 workouts per week—as well as the intensity, pace, and overall volume of work, for both the upper and lower body as well as the core. Be sure you have read all of the general program guidelines and safety tips in 60-Second Essentials, as well as the Dripping Sweat–specific guidelines that follow.

WORKOUT GUIDELINES

Disclaimer: It is strongly advised that you consult your physician prior to beginning this or any other exercise or nutrition program. A complete physical examination is highly recommended if you are sedentary, have high cholesterol, have high blood pressure, have diabetes, are overweight, or are over 30 years old.

- Work out 4 days per week, alternating between the A and B workouts (you'll perform each workout twice during the week).

- "20 on, 10 off" means you will work very hard for 20 seconds, followed by a period of rest for 10 seconds.

- Do not skip the warm-up routine outlined in this program!

- Don't train to failure/exhaustion. You should be able to do 1 more rep at the end of each set. If you can't, reduce the amount of weight you are using.

- If your time is limited, reduce the number of sets in the workout but do not, under any circumstances, skip the warm-up.

WEEKLY SCHEDULE	
Day 1	Workout A
Day 2	Recovery Day
Day 3	Workout B
Day 4	Recovery Day
Day 5	Workout A
Day 6	Recovery Day
Day 7	Workout B*

*You will follow this day with workout A the very next day,
so you will be working out on consecutive days in this advanced phase.

WARM-UP

Complete the 10 exercises below, resting only as long as it takes to transition between exercises.

EXERCISE	REPS	REST
Side-Lying Rotation (page 62)	6 reps/side	
Glute Bridge (page 64)	10 reps	
Quad/Hip Flexor Mobilization* (page 66)	6 reps/side	
Half-Kneeling Groin Mobilization (page 68)	6 reps/side	
Cat/Camel Drill (page 70)	10 rcps	
Bird Dog (page 72)	6 reps/side	
Arm Circles (page 78)	10 reps each direction	
Arm Crosses (page 80)	10 reps	
Chest Stretch (page 74)	20 seconds/side	
Lat Stretch (page 76)	20 seconds/side	

WORKOUT A

WORKOUT CIRCUIT #1

Repeat 4 times with a 15-second rest between exercises. Rest 45 seconds between circuits.

	EXERCISE	REPS	REST
	Dumbbell Romanian Deadlift (page 172)	12 reps	15 seconds rest/transition
	Dumbbell Pullover (page 134)	12 reps	15 seconds rest/transition
	Stability Ball Leg Curl (page 170)	12 reps	15 seconds rest/transition
	Long Lever Plank (page 182)	30 seconds	

WORKOUT CIRCUIT #2

Repeat 4 times with a 15-second rest between exercises. Rest 45 seconds between circuits.

	EXERCISE	REPS	REST
	3-Point Dumbbell Row (page 126)	10 reps/side	15 seconds rest/transition
	Single-Leg Hip Thrust (page 168)	8 reps/side	15 seconds rest/transition
	Bent-Over Band Lat Pulldown (page 132)	8 reps/side	15 seconds rest/transition
	Tall Kneeling Band Core Press (page 210)	5 reps/side (Hold for 5 seconds in the arms extended position.)	

WORKOUT CIRCUIT #3

Repeat 3 times with a 15-second rest between exercises. Rest 45 seconds between circuits.

EXERCISE	REPS	REST
Power Band Row (page 122)	12 reps	15 seconds rest/transition
Prone Cobra (page 176)	12 reps	15 seconds rest/transition
Bent-Over Dumbbell Rear-Deltoid Raise (page 128)	12 reps	15 seconds rest/transition
Hollow Body Hold (hands behind head) (page 194)	30 seconds	

METABOLIC BLAST CIRCUIT

EXERCISE	REPS	REST
Run in Place (page 216)	20 on/10 off x 4 rounds	45 seconds rest
Cross-Body Mountain Climber (page 236)	20 on/10 off x 4 rounds	45 seconds rest
Side-to-Side Shuffle (5 yards each direction) (page 220)	20 on/10 off x 4 rounds	

WORKOUT B

WORKOUT CIRCUIT #1

Repeat 4 times with a 15-second rest between exercises. Rest 45 seconds between circuits.

	EXERCISE	REPS	REST
	Piston Push-Up OR Piston Bench Push-Up* (pages 90, 92)	10 reps	15 seconds rest/transition
	Goblet Combination Lunge (page 160)	10 reps/side	15 seconds rest/transition
	Dumbbell Iron Cross (page 114)	30 seconds	15 seconds rest/transition
	Inch Worm (page 184)	4 reps (out and back is one rep)	

*Your choice here depends on your fitness level. The first time you do this workout, experiment with both variations over the 4 sets to determine which one is both challenging yet doable.

WORKOUT CIRCUIT #2

Repeat 4 times with a 15-second rest between exercises. Rest 45 seconds between circuits.

	EXERCISE	REPS	REST
	Dumbbell Push Press (page 108)	10 reps	15 seconds rest/transition
	2-Stage Dumbbell Goblet Squat (page 138)	8 reps	15 seconds rest/transition
	Incline Dumbbell Chest Fly (page 104)	12 reps	15 seconds rest/transition
	Double-Arm Dumbbell Carry (page 190)	40 steps	

WORKOUT CIRCUIT #3

Repeat 3 times with a 15-second rest between exercises. Rest 45 seconds between circuits.

	EXERCISE	REPS	REST
	Wall Sit (page 146)	30 seconds	15 seconds rest/transition
	Jump Squat (page 144)	8 reps	15 seconds rest/transition
	Power Dumbbell Front Raise (page 116)	12 reps	15 seconds rest/transition
	Stability Ball Crunch (page 198)	12 reps	

METABOLIC BLAST CIRCUIT

	EXERCISE	REPS	REST
	Short Shuttle Run (5 yards each direction) (page 222)	20 on/10 off x 4 rounds	45 seconds rest
	Dumbbell Swing (page 230)	20 on/10 off x 4 rounds	45 seconds rest
	Phantom Rope Skipping (page 218)	20 on/10 off x 4 rounds	

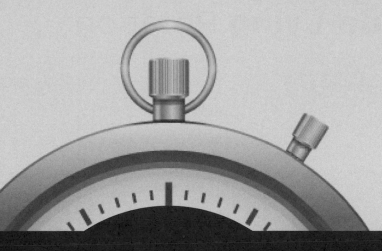

PART III

60 SECOND SWEAT EXERCISES

Side-Lying Rotation

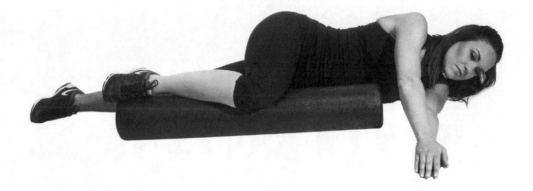

1. Lie on your left side with your right hip flexed and your right knee bent. Your arms should be straight out in front of you with your palms together.

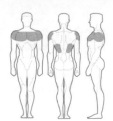

WHAT IT DOES:
Loosens up your
mid back, chest, and
shoulders.

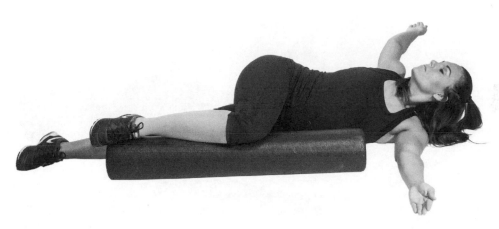

2. Rotate through the middle of your back, opening up your chest and right arm in an arching motion, until your right hand nearly touches the floor on the opposite side.

3. Rotate back to the starting position and repeat for the suggested number of reps. Repeat on the other side, flexing the left hip and left knee.

FORM TIP: Really focus on moving through your mid back and keeping your lower back out of the exercise.

Glute Bridge

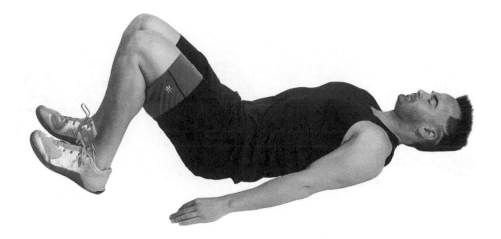

1. Lie flat on your back with your knees bent at 90 degrees, your heels on the floor, and your feet flexed.

WHAT IT DOES:
Activates your rear end and hamstrings and lengthens the front of your hips.

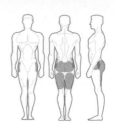

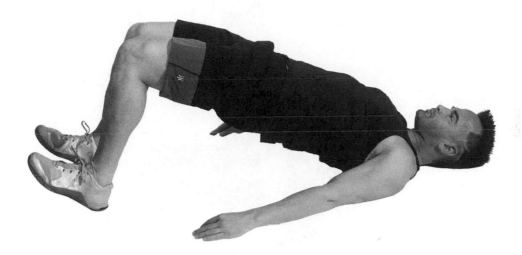

2. Drive through your heels to push your hips up to form a bridge. Your knees, hips, and shoulders should form a straight line. Focus on squeezing your rear end in the top position before lowering back to the floor. Repeat for the suggested number of reps.

FORM TIP: Avoid bridging up too high and hyperextending your lower back.

Quad/Hip **Flexor Mobilization**

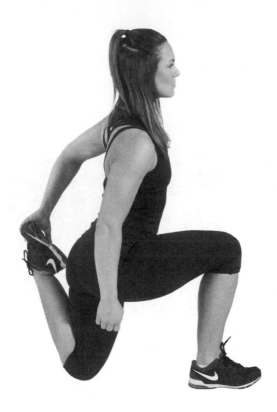

1. Assume a half-kneeling position with your left knee on the ground and your right leg out in front of you bent at 90 degrees. Keeping an upright posture, grab your left ankle with your left hand and slowly pull your left heel toward your rear end.

WHAT IT DOES:
Stretches and lengthens the front of your hip and thigh.

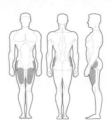

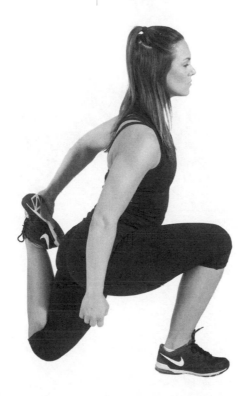

2. Slowly shift your weight forward slightly until you feel a gentle pull in the front of your left thigh and the front of your left hip before transitioning back to the starting position.

3. Continue moving in and out for the suggested number of reps. Repeat with your right knee down and your left leg out.

FORM TIP: Before starting the movement, draw your rib cage down by tilting your hip bones back.

Half-Kneeling
Groin Mobilization

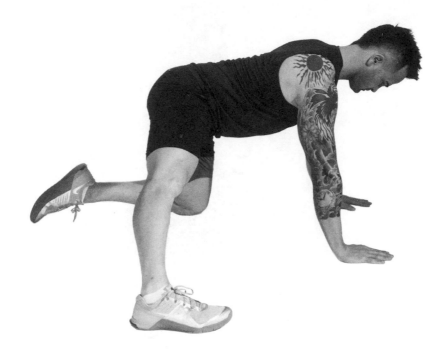

1. Get on your hands and knees with your wrists under your shoulders and your knees under your hips.

2. Extend your right leg out to the side, keeping the knee straight and your foot flat on the floor.

WHAT IT DOES:
Stretches and
lengthens the muscles on
the inside of
your thigh.

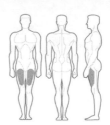

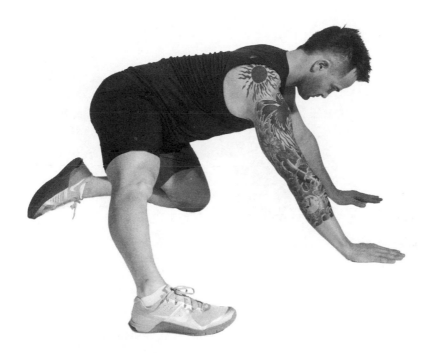

3. Slowly rock back toward the left heel until you feel a stretch in your right groin on the inside of your thigh.

4. Slowly rock back to the starting position. Continue in this manner, rocking back and forth for the suggested number of reps, before switching to the left leg.

FORM TIP: Keep your back perfectly flat. Your neck should form a straight line with your back.

Cat/Camel Drill

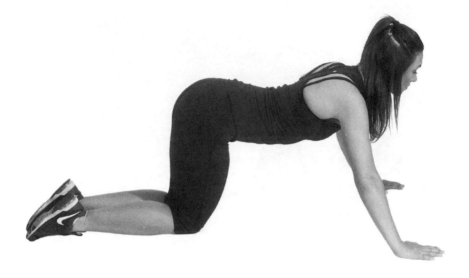

1. Get on your hands and knees with your wrists under your shoulders and your knees under your hips.

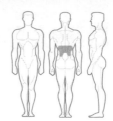

WHAT IT DOES:
Loosens up your
lower back.

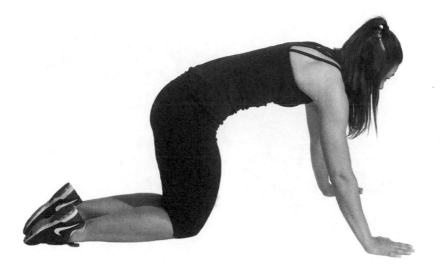

2. Slowly arch up, rolling your hip bones toward your chin, making a "C" shape out of your spine.

3. Return to the starting position by allowing your spine to flatten back out. Continue in this manner, arching up and down, for the suggested number of reps.

FORM TIP: When coming back down to the starting position, stop at a neutral flat-back position. Do not hyperextend your lower back.

Bird Dog

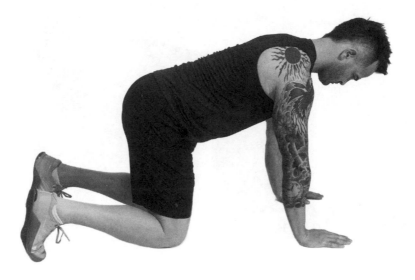

1. Get on your hands and knees with your wrists under your shoulders and your knees under your hips.

WHAT IT DOES:
Activates your rear end and rear shoulder muscles as well as creating core stability and control.

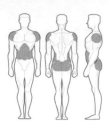

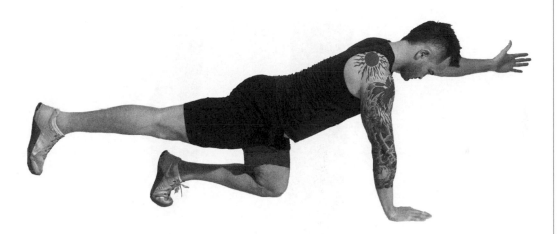

2. Keeping your abdominals tight, slowly extend your left arm out in front of you, rotating your thumb up, as you simultaneously extend your right leg behind you. Pause in the extended position for a full second before returning to the starting position. Repeat for the suggested number of reps before switching sides.

FORM TIP: Perform this exercise deliberately and slowly. Do not allow your torso and hips to tip or rotate to either side. They should remain parallel to the floor.

Chest Stretch

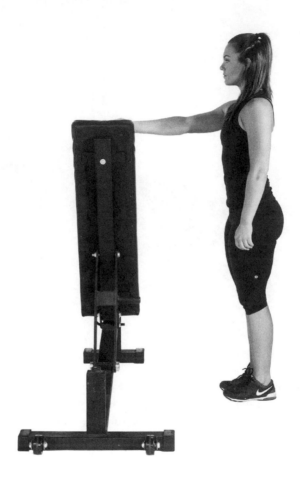

1. Standing at arm's length away, grab a secure surface (an upright bench, a door frame, or a post) with your right arm at shoulder level.

2. Rotate your torso and hips away from the secure surface and step out slightly with your left foot until you feel a moderate stretch through your right chest muscle.

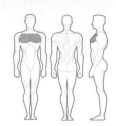

WHAT IT DOES:
Stretches and lengthens your chest muscles.

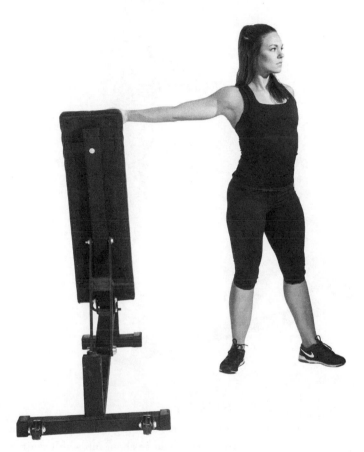

3. Hold the stretch for the suggested amount of time before switching to the left side.

FORM TIP: To avoid injuring your shoulder, think about "packing" your shoulder blade into your spine on the stretched side.

Lat Stretch

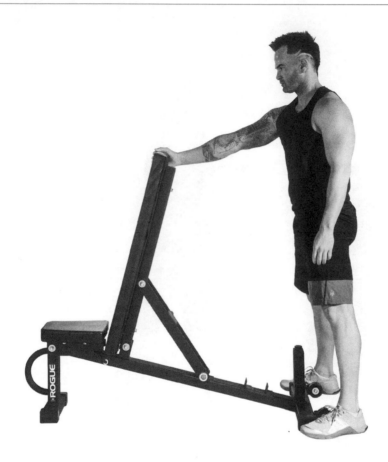

1. Standing an arm's length away, grab a secure surface (an upright bench, a door frame, or a post) with your right arm at shoulder level. Your feet should be about hip width apart.

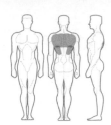

WHAT IT DOES:
Stretches and lengthens the muscles in your upper and mid back.

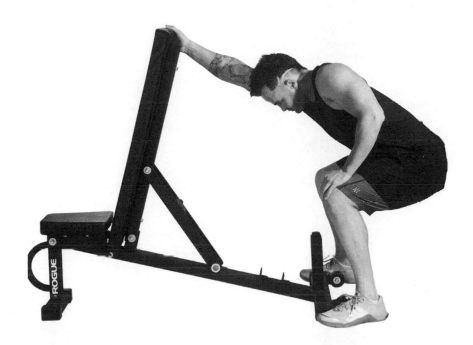

2. Slowly sink your hips down and back until you feel a mild stretch in the muscles under your armpit and the big muscles running along the side of your spine. Let your head and upper body bend forward toward the secure surface.

3. Hold the stretch for the suggested amount of time before switching to the left side.

FORM TIP: Breathe deeply to enhance the stretch.

Arm Circles

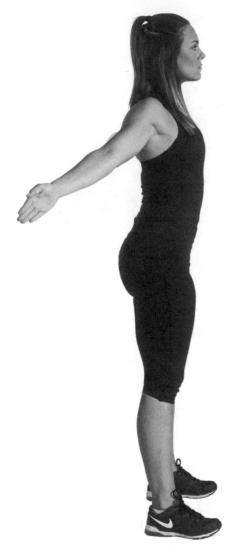

1. Holding your arms out to the side at shoulder level with the elbows straight, slowly make small clockwise circles rotating from your shoulders.

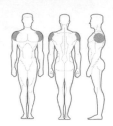

WHAT IT DOES:
Loosens up your
shoulders.

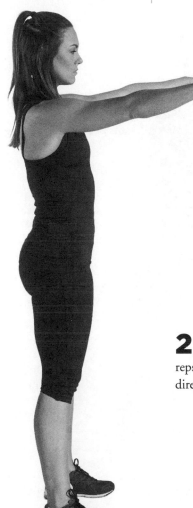

2. Perform for the suggested number of reps before switching to a counterclockwise direction for an identical number of reps.

FORM TIP: Gradually increase the size of the circles throughout the set.

Arm Crosses

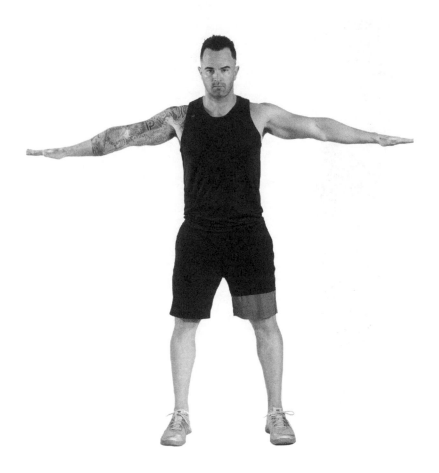

1. Stand with your feet hip width apart and your arms out to the side at shoulder level, with the elbows straight.

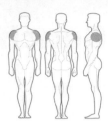

WHAT IT DOES:
Loosens up your
shoulders.

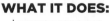

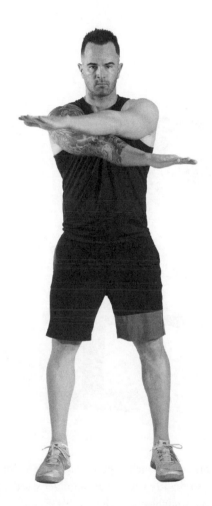

2. Move your arms inward and make an "X" motion, crossing your arms in front of your chest.

3. Bring the arms back out to the starting position, and continue crossing the arms in and out for the suggested number of reps.

FORM TIP: Start slowly, and gradually pick up the speed of the exercise.

Bench Push-Up

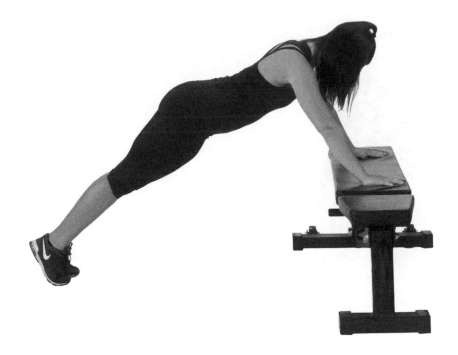

1. Assume a push-up position with your hands on a flat bench slightly wider than shoulder width apart and the balls of your feet on the floor, also slightly wider than shoulder width apart. Your back should be flat, and your neck should form a straight line with your back.

2. Keeping your abdominals and rear end tight, slowly lower yourself toward the bench until your chest touches or nearly touches the bench, allowing your arms to tuck in slightly toward your sides.

WHAT IT DOES:
Strengthens the muscles in your chest, the front of your shoulders, the back of your arms, and your core.

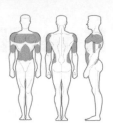

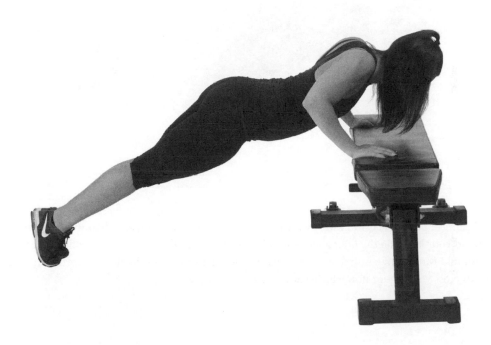

3. Push back up to the starting position, and repeat for the suggested number of reps.

FORM TIP: If you have trouble touching your chest to the bench for the required number of reps, adjust your range of motion and don't lower yourself down quite as far.

Kneeling Push-Up

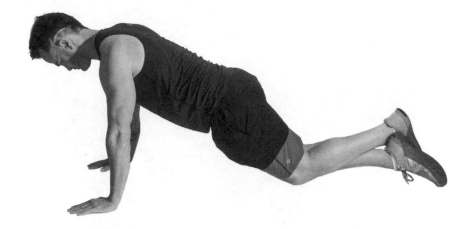

1. Assume a push-up position with your hands on the floor slightly wider than shoulder width apart and your knees on the floor about shoulder width apart. Your back should be flat, and your neck should form a straight line with your back. Your feet can be on the floor or in the air, and you can cross your legs or not, whichever is more comfortable.

WHAT IT DOES:
Strengthens the muscles in your chest, the front of your shoulders, the back of your arms, and your core.

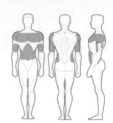

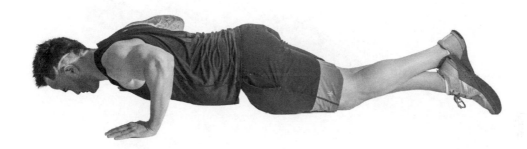

2. Keeping your abdominals and rear end tight, slowly lower yourself toward the floor until your chest touches or nearly touches the floor, allowing your arms to tuck in slightly toward your sides.

3. Push back up to the starting position, and repeat for the suggested number of reps.

FORM TIP: If you have trouble touching your chest to the floor for the required number of reps, adjust your range of motion and don't lower yourself down quite as far.

Push-Up

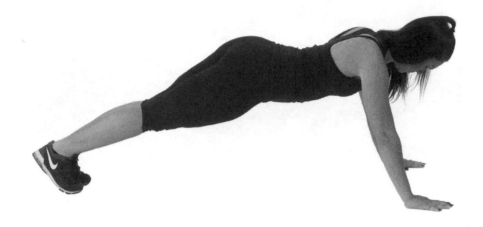

1. Assume a push-up position with your hands on the floor slightly wider than shoulder width apart and the balls of your feet about shoulder width apart. Your back should be flat, and your neck should form a straight line with your back.

WHAT IT DOES:
Strengthens the muscles
in your chest, the front
of your shoulders,
the back of your arms,
and your core.

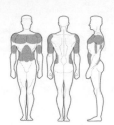

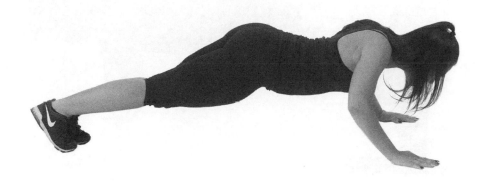

2. Keeping your abdominals and rear end tight, slowly lower yourself toward the floor until your chest touches or nearly touches the floor, allowing your arms to tuck in slightly toward your sides.

3. Push back up to the starting position, and repeat for the suggested number of reps.

FORM TIP: If you have trouble touching your chest to the floor for the required number of reps, you are not ready for this exercise. Instead, do Bench or Kneeling Push-Ups.

Feet-Elevated Push-Up

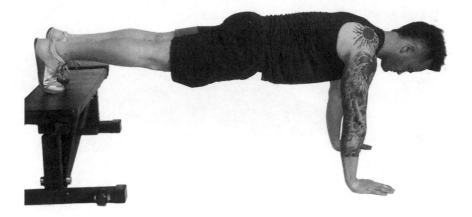

1. Assume a push-up position with your hands on the floor slightly wider than shoulder width apart and the balls of your feet on a flat bench about shoulder width apart. Your back should be flat, and your neck should form a straight line with your back.

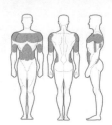

WHAT IT DOES:
Strengthens the muscles
in your chest, the front
of your shoulders,
the back of your arms,
and your core.

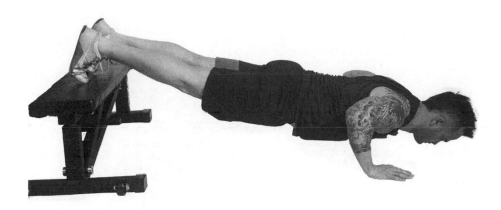

2. Keeping your abdominals and rear end tight, slowly lower yourself toward the floor until your chest touches or nearly touches the floor, allowing your arms to tuck in slightly toward your sides.

3. Push back up to the staring position and repeat for the suggested number of reps.

FORM TIP: Don't let your hips sag. If you have trouble touching your chest to the floor for the suggested number of reps, you are not ready for this exercise. Instead, do Push-Ups.

Piston Bench Push-Up

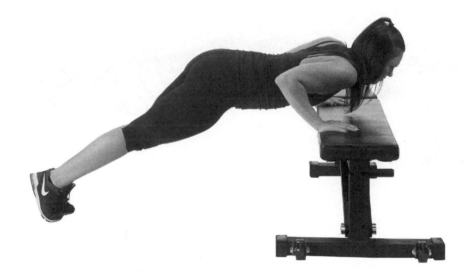

1. Assume a push-up position with your hands on a flat bench slightly more than shoulder width apart and the balls of your feet on the floor about shoulder width apart. Your back should be flat, and your neck should form a straight line with your back.

2. Keeping your abdominals and rear end tight, slowly lower yourself until your chest touches or nearly touches the bench, allowing your arms to tuck in slightly toward your sides.

WHAT IT DOES:
Strengthens your entire core and the muscles in your chest, the front of your shoulders, and the back of your arms.

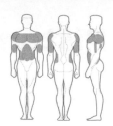

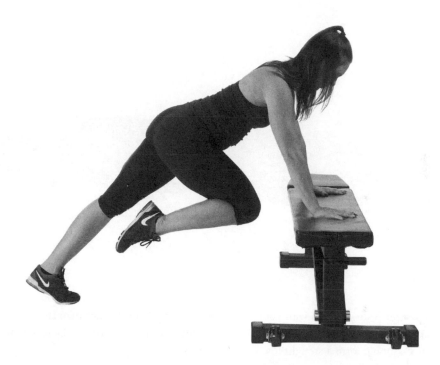

3. Push back up while simultaneously flexing your right hip and driving your right knee toward your right shoulder.

4. Lower back down and repeat with the opposite leg. Continue in this fashion, alternating legs, for the suggested number of reps.

FORM TIP: Come to a complete pause and check your form between reps; do not rush through this exercise.

Piston Push-Up

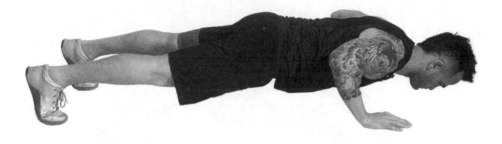

1. Assume a push-up position with your hands on the floor slightly wider than shoulder width apart and the balls of your feet on the floor about shoulder width apart. Your back should be flat, and your neck should form a straight line with your back.

2. Keeping your abdominals and rear end tight, slowly lower yourself toward the floor until your chest touches or nearly touches the floor, allowing your arms to tuck in slightly toward your sides.

WHAT IT DOES:
Strengthens the muscles
in your chest, the front
of your shoulders,
the back of your arms,
and your core.

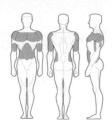

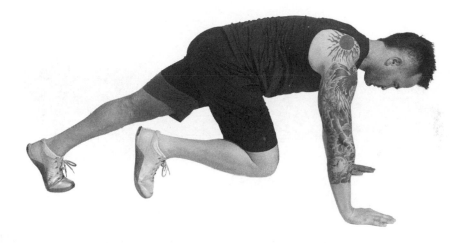

3. Drive your hands through the floor and push back up while simultaneously driving your right knee toward your right elbow.

4. Lower back down and repeat with the opposite leg. Continue in this fashion, alternating legs, for the suggested number of reps.

FORM TIP: To avoid irritating your lower back and taking emphasis off your abdominals, don't let your hips sag.

T-Rotation Push-Up

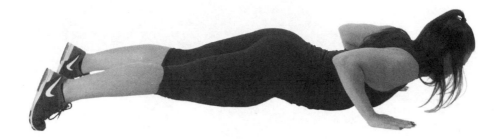

1. Assume a push-up position with your hands on the floor slightly wider than shoulder width apart and the balls of your feet on the floor slightly wider than hip width apart. Your back should be flat, and your neck should form a straight line with your back.

2. Keeping your abdominals and rear end tight, slowly lower yourself toward the floor until your chest touches or nearly touches the floor, allowing your arms to tuck in slightly toward your sides.

3. Drive your hands through the floor and push back up while simultaneously rotating to your right. Open up your right arm overhead and pivot onto the sides of your feet, balancing on your left hand, while you drive your right hip up. Both arms should be straight, creating a "T" with your body.

WHAT IT DOES:
Strengthens the muscles
in your chest, the front
of your shoulders,
the back of your arms,
and your core.

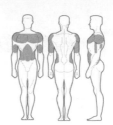

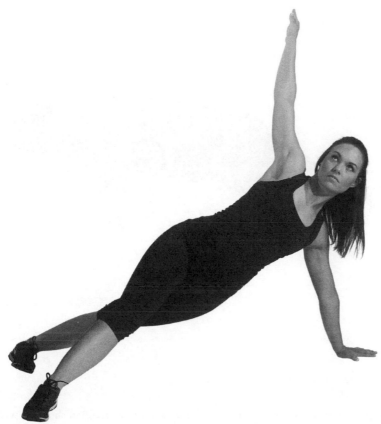

4. Pause for one second in this position before rotating back onto the balls of your feet and placing your right hand back on the floor into the push-up position. Repeat for the suggested number of reps before switching sides and opening up to your left for an identical number of reps.

FORM TIP: As you open up and rotate, really emphasize driving your hip up into the air to maximize the core strengthening effect of this exercise.

T-Rotation

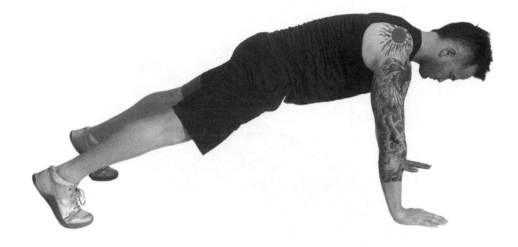

1. Assume a push-up position with your hands on the floor slightly wider than shoulder width apart and the balls of your feet on the floor slightly wider than hip width apart. Your back should be flat, and your neck should form a straight line with your back.

2. Rotate to your right, opening up your right arm overhead and pivoting onto the sides of your feet. Balance on your left hand while driving your right hip up. Both arms should be straight, creating a "T" with your body.

WHAT IT DOES:
Strengthens the
core and increases
shoulder stability.

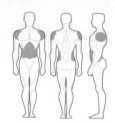

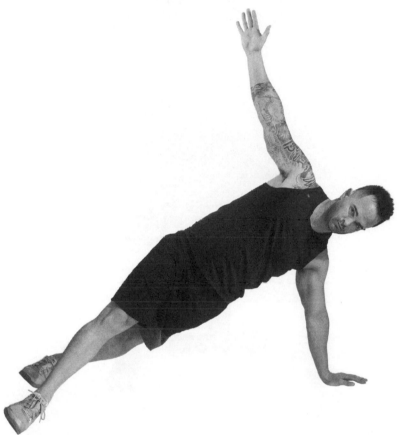

3. Pause for a full second in the open position before rotating back in and onto the balls of your feet and placing your right hand back on the floor into the push-up position. Repeat for the suggested number of reps before switching sides and opening up to your left for an identical number of reps.

FORM TIP: Because of the complexity of this exercise, do not rush.

Flat Dumbbell Chest Press

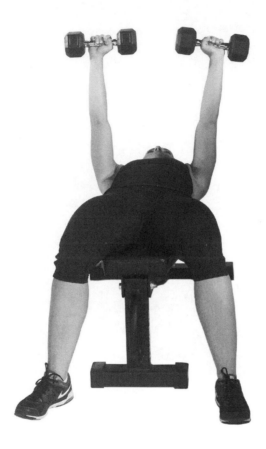

1. Lie on your back on a flat bench with your feet firmly on the floor and your arms extended over your chest, holding a dumbbell in each hand. Your palms should face forward.

2. Slowly bend your arms to lower the dumbbells down and outward until they are on either side of your chest.

WHAT IT DOES:
Strengthens the muscles in your chest, the front of your shoulders, and the back of your arms.

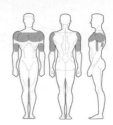

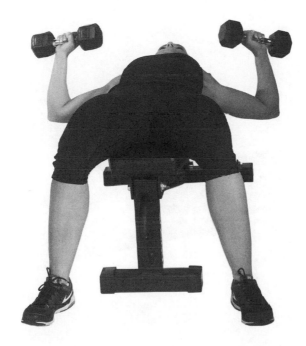

3. Extend your arms straight up and over your chest again, pressing back up to the starting position. Pause briefly at the top before repeating for the suggested number of reps.

FORM TIP: Don't lower the dumbbells too deep, or you'll risk injuring your shoulders. You should feel a nice stretch in your chest and still be able to see your knuckles and thumbs in the bottom position.

Incline Dumbbell Chest Press

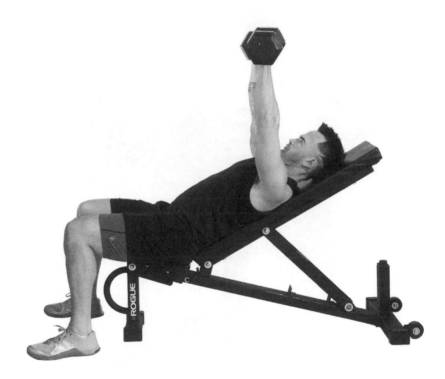

1. Lie on your back on an incline bench set to 45 degrees with your feet firmly on the floor and your arms extended over your chest, holding a dumbbell in each hand. Your palms should face forward.

2. Slowly bend your arms to lower the dumbbells down and outward until they are on either side of your chest.

WHAT IT DOES:
Strengthens the muscles in your chest, the front of your shoulders, and the back of your arms.

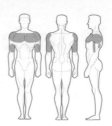

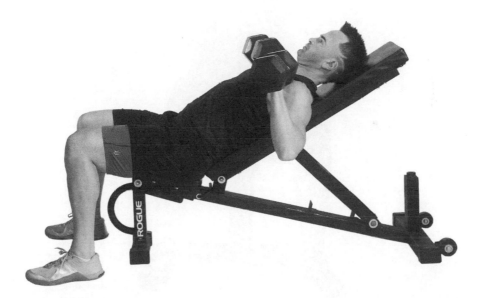

3. Extend your arms straight up and over your chest again, pressing back up to the starting position. Pause briefly at the top before repeating for the suggested number of reps.

FORM TIP: Don't lower the dumbbells too deep, or you'll risk injuring your shoulders. You should feel a nice stretch in your chest and still be able to see your knuckles and thumbs.

Dumbbell Crush Press

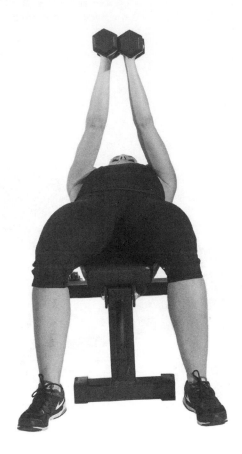

1. Lie on your back on a flat bench with your feet firmly on the floor and your arms extended over your chest, holding a dumbbell in each hand. Turn your hands in so your palms are facing, to "crush" the dumbbells up against each other.

2. Pushing the dumbbells together, slowly bend your arms to lower the dumbbells down just to the middle of your chest.

WHAT IT DOES:
Strengthens the muscles in your chest, the front of your shoulders, and the back of your arms.

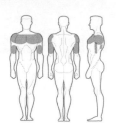

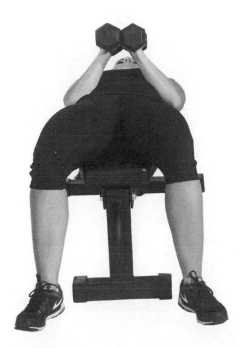

3. Extend your arms straight up and over your chest again, pressing back up to the starting position. Pause briefly at the top before repeating for the suggested number of reps.

FORM TIP: Make sure you keep pushing the dumbbells together during both the lowering and lifting phases, as this increases the demand on the target muscles.

Incline Dumbbell Chest Fly

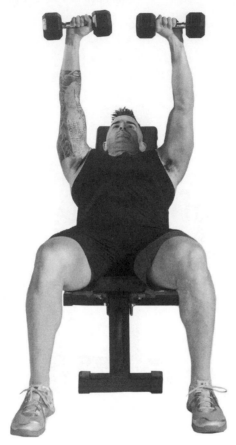

1. Lie on your back on an incline bench set to 45 degrees, with your feet firmly on the floor and your arms extended over your chest, holding a dumbbell in each hand. Your palms should face forward.

2. Keeping your palms facing forward and your elbows soft, slowly lower the dumbbells down in an arching motion until you feel a gentle stretch in your chest muscles.

WHAT IT DOES:
Strengthens the
muscles in your chest.

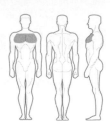

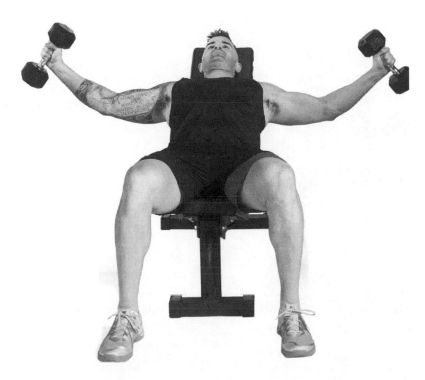

3. Smoothly raise the dumbbells back to the starting position in the reverse motion, and repeat for the suggested number of reps.

FORM TIP: Keep your palms facing forward, rather than facing each other, to better work your chest muscles. Think about hugging a large barrel or beach ball sitting on your chest during the lifting phase.

Seated Dumbbell
Shoulder Press

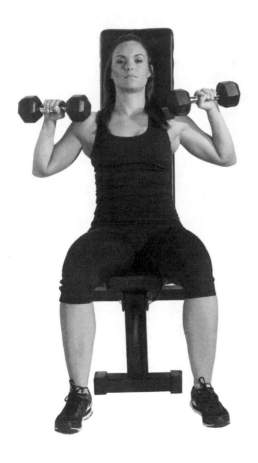

1. Sit on a bench with the back pad angled to a completely upright position at 90 degrees, with your feet planted firmly on the floor. Hold a dumbbell in each hand at shoulder level with your elbows out and your palms facing forward.

WHAT IT DOES:
Strengthens the muscles in the front of your shoulders and the back of your arms.

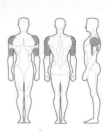

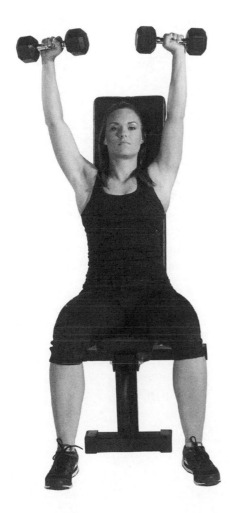

2. Press the dumbbells upward until they are directly overhead and your arms are fully extended.

3. Pause for a full second in the overhead position before lowering the dumbbells back down to the starting position. Repeat for the suggested number of reps.

FORM TIP: If you find this exercise causes any shoulder discomfort, bring your elbows in and allow your palms to face each other.

Dumbbell Push Press

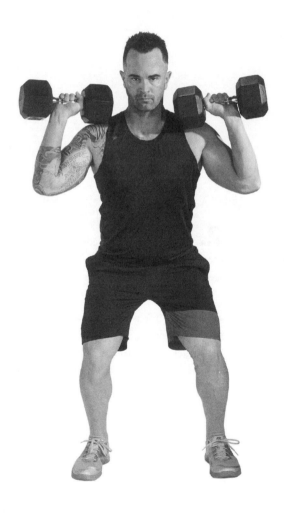

1. Stand with your feet slightly wider than shoulder width apart. Hold a dumbbell in each hand at shoulder level, with your elbows out and your palms facing forward.

2. Bend your knees and lower yourself down about 6 inches into a quarter squat.

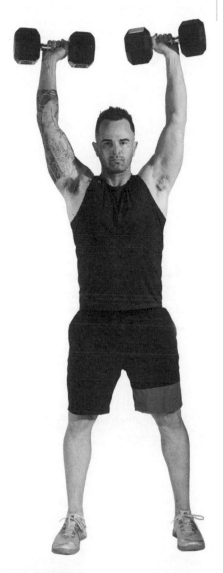

WHAT IT DOES:
Strengthens the muscles in the front of your shoulders and the back of your arms while building total-body power and explosiveness.

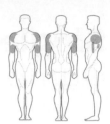

3. Explosively—with as much force as possible—press the dumbbells overhead by extending your arms, pushing your feet down into the floor, pushing your hips forward, and straightening your legs.

4. Pause in the overhead position for a full second before lowering the dumbbells slowly back down to shoulder level.

5. Take a full second to check your form before repeating for the suggested number of reps.

FORM TIP: Focus on snapping your hips explosively—with as much force as possible—during the lifting phase.

Single-Arm
Dumbell Push Press

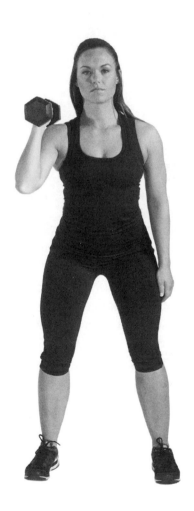

1. Stand with your feet slightly wider than shoulder width apart. Hold a dumbbell in your right hand at shoulder level, with your elbow out and your palm facing in. Let your left arm hang by your side.

2. Bend your knees and lower yourself down about 6 inches into a quarter squat.

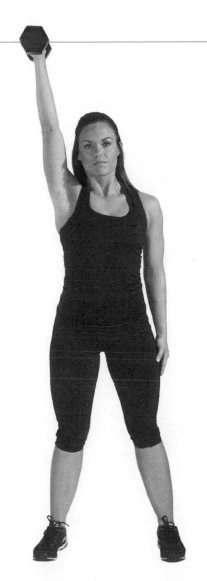

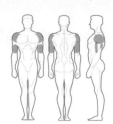

WHAT IT DOES:
Strengthens the muscles in the front of your shoulders and the back of your arms, while building total-body power and explosiveness.

3. Explosively—with as much force as possible—press the dumbbell overhead by extending your arms, pushing your feet hard into the floor, pushing your hips forward, and straightening your legs.

4. Pause in the overhead position for a full second before lowering the dumbbell slowly back down to shoulder level.

5. Take a full second to check your form before repeating for the suggested number of reps, and then switch to the left side.

FORM TIP: Keep your core tight, and do not allow the weight of the dumbbell to bend you laterally to the side. If it helps your balance, you can put your left arm out to your side.

Dumbbell Thruster

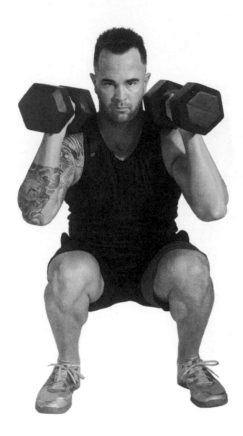

1. Stand with your feet about hip width apart. Hold a dumbbell in each hand, resting the dumbbells lightly on your shoulders as if in a rack, with your elbows pointed slightly up and your palms facing in.

2. Keeping an upright posture and not allowing the dumbbells to tip down, bend your knees and lower yourself down into a full squat, with your thighs below parallel to the floor, as low as you can comfortably go.

WHAT IT DOES:
Strengthens the muscles in the front of your shoulders, the back of your arms, and your hips and thighs, while building total-body power and explosiveness.

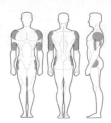

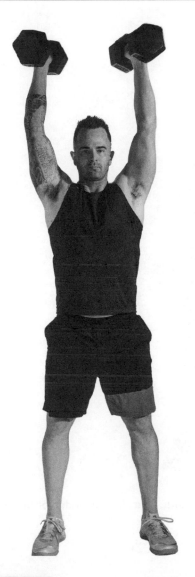

3. Explosively—with as much force as possible—stand back up and press the dumbbells over your head until your arms are fully extended, keeping your palms facing in.

4. Return the dumbbells to the starting position. Take a full second to check your form before repeating for the suggested number of reps.

FORM TIP: You may have heard that in a full squat, the back of your thighs should touch your calves. But if you have any tightness in your joints, you may not be able to get that low. Don't force it; just go as low as you comfortably can.

Dumbbell Iron Cross

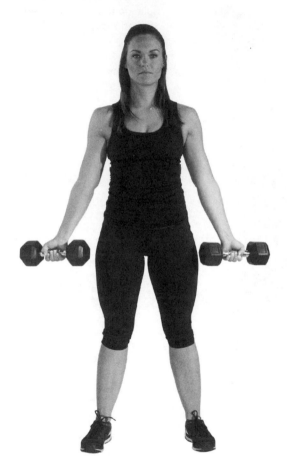

1. Stand with your feet slightly wider than shoulder width apart, holding a dumbbell in each hand at your sides with the palms facing forward.

WHAT IT DOES:
Strengthens the
muscles in the sides
of your shoulders
and upper back.

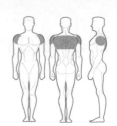

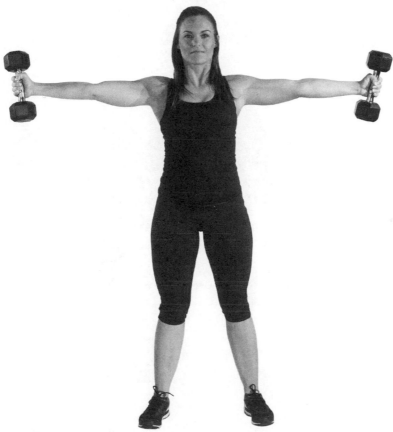

2. Raise your arms out to the sides to shoulder level, creating a cross with your body. Your palms should remain facing forward.

3. Hold this position for the suggested amount of time.

FORM TIP: Start with a very conservative weight on this exercise. If you cannot maintain the cross position for the suggested amount of time, reduce the weight you are using.

Power Dumbbell Front Raise

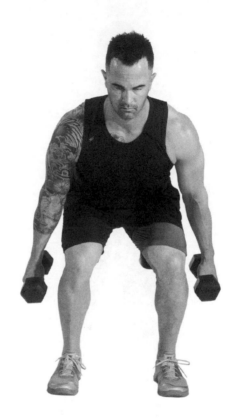

1. Stand with your feet about shoulder width apart while holding a dumbbell in each hand, palms facing in toward your thighs.

2. Bend your knees, leaning slightly forward, and lower yourself down about 6 inches into a quarter squat.

3. Explosively—with as much force as possible—push your hips forward, straighten your legs, and raise the dumbbells in front of you until they are completely over your head, keeping your elbows straight and palms facing in.

WHAT IT DOES:
Strengthens the muscles in the front of your shoulders, while building total-body power and explosiveness.

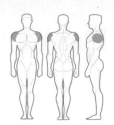

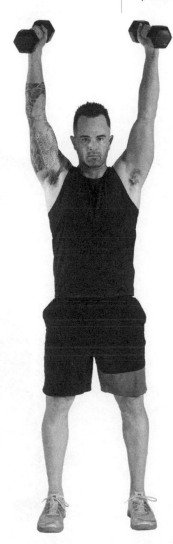

4. Pause for a full second in the overhead position before lowering the dumbbells back slowly to the starting position and immediately lowering yourself back into the quarter squat. Repeat for the suggested number of reps.

FORM TIP: Except when you pause in the overhead position, you should be moving constantly through this exercise; find a rhythm to keep the movement fluid.

Band Row

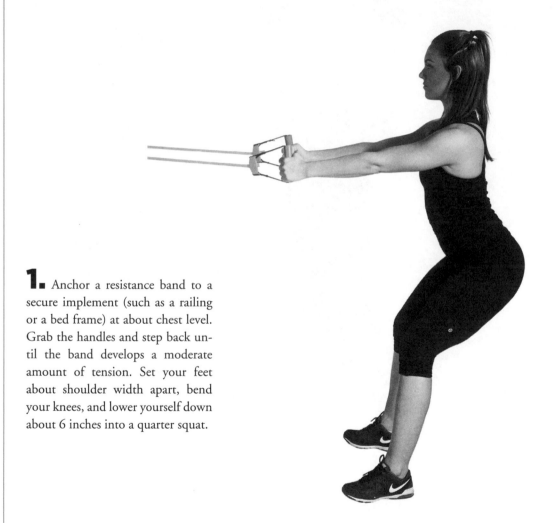

1. Anchor a resistance band to a secure implement (such as a railing or a bed frame) at about chest level. Grab the handles and step back until the band develops a moderate amount of tension. Set your feet about shoulder width apart, bend your knees, and lower yourself down about 6 inches into a quarter squat.

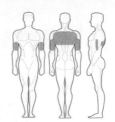

WHAT IT DOES:
Strengthens the muscles in your upper back and the front of your arms.

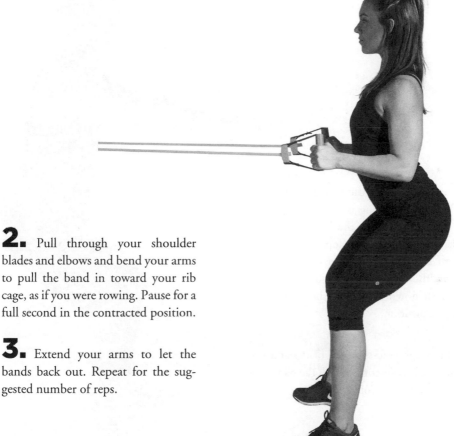

2. Pull through your shoulder blades and elbows and bend your arms to pull the band in toward your rib cage, as if you were rowing. Pause for a full second in the contracted position.

3. Extend your arms to let the bands back out. Repeat for the suggested number of reps.

FORM TIP: When rowing the band in, think about drawing your shoulder blades together.

Alternating Band Row

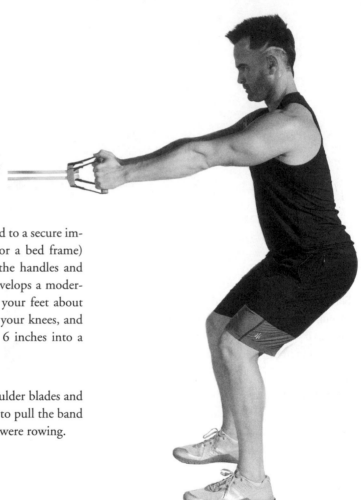

1. Anchor a resistance band to a secure implement (such as a railing or a bed frame) at about chest level. Grab the handles and step back until the band develops a moderate amount of tension. Set your feet about shoulder width apart, bend your knees, and lower yourself down about 6 inches into a quarter squat position.

2. Pull through your shoulder blades and elbows and bend your arms to pull the band into your rib cage, as if you were rowing.

WHAT IT DOES:
Strengthens the muscles in your upper back and the front of your arms.

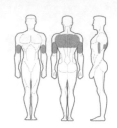

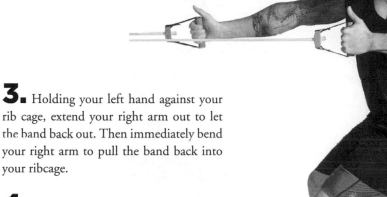

3. Holding your left hand against your rib cage, extend your right arm out to let the band back out. Then immediately bend your right arm to pull the band back into your ribcage.

4. Switch arms. Holding your right hand against your rib cage, extend your left arm out to let the band back out. Then immediately bend your left arm to pull the band back in toward your rib cage.

5. Continue alternating arms for the suggested number of reps on each arm.

FORM TIP: When rowing the band in, think about drawing your shoulder blades together.

Power Band Row

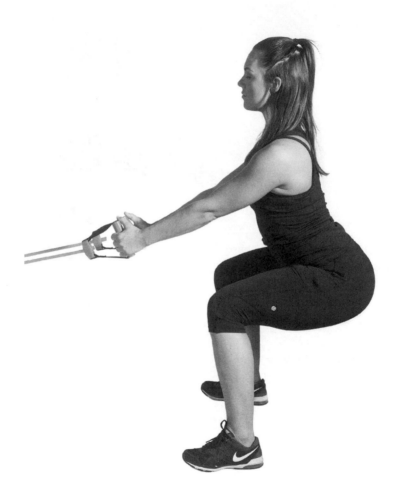

1. Anchor a resistance band to a secure implement (such as a railing or a bed frame) at about chest level. Grab the handles and step back until the band develops a moderate amount of tension. Set your feet about shoulder width apart, bend your knees, and lower yourself down into a half squat, with your thighs parallel to the floor.

WHAT IT DOES:
Strengthens the muscles in your upper back and the front of your arms, while developing full-body power and explosiveness.

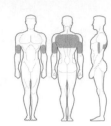

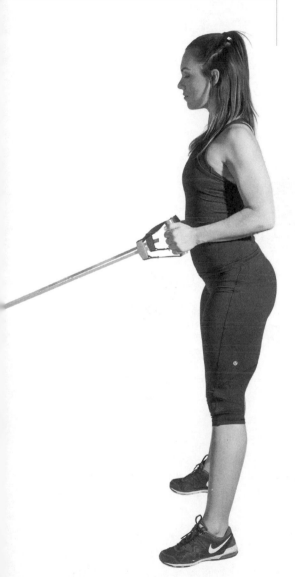

2. Explosively—with as much force as possible—push your hips forward and straighten your legs while simultaneously pulling through your shoulder blades and elbows and bending your arms to pull the band in toward your rib cage, as if you were rowing.

3. Immediately squat back down to the starting position while simultaneously extending your arms to let the band back out. Repeat for the suggested number of reps.

FORM TIP: Focus on coordinating the movement of your arms and legs. Your arms should be extending as you go down into the squat, and your legs should be fully straightened as your hands come in toward your ribs.

Chest-Supported
Dumbbell Row

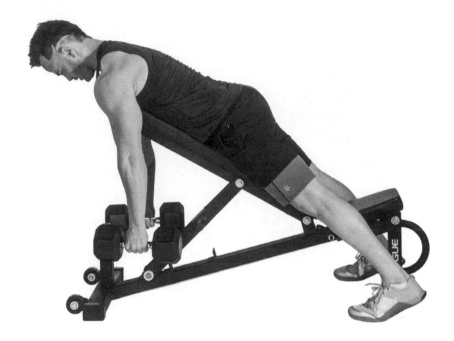

1. Set an incline bench to about a 45-degree angle and lie facedown with your head and upper chest hanging off the end of the bench. Hold a dumbbell in each hand and let your arms hang straight down with your palms facing each other.

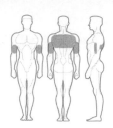

WHAT IT DOES:
Strengthens the
muscles in your upper
back and the front of
your arms.

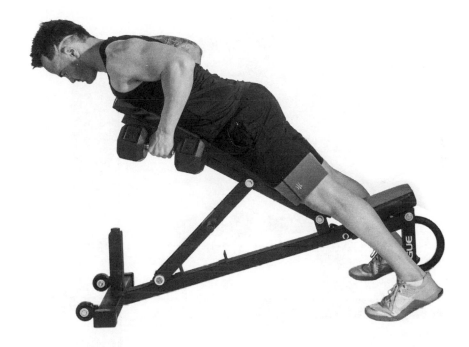

2. Keeping your chest firmly on the bench pad, pull through your shoulder blades and elbows, and bend your arms to row the dumbbells up until they meet the bench.

3. Extend your arms to lower the dumbbells back down to the starting position, and repeat for the suggested number of reps.

FORM TIP: Make sure your chest stays flat and secure against the bench; don't use your lower back.

3-Point Dumbbell Row

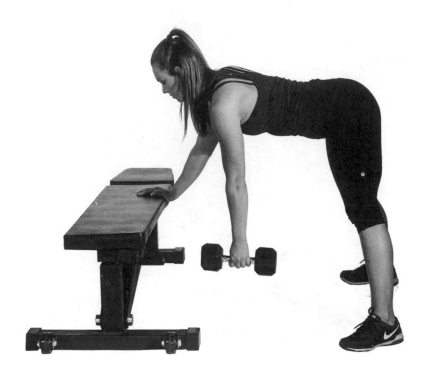

1. Stand alongside a flat bench with your feet about hip width apart. Bend from the waist and plant your right hand on the bench. Your right hand and two feet form the 3 points. Hold a dumbbell in your left hand and let your arm hang straight down. Your back should be flat, and your neck should form a straight line with your back.

WHAT IT DOES:
Strengthens the muscles in your upper back and the front of your arms.

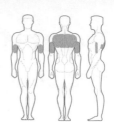

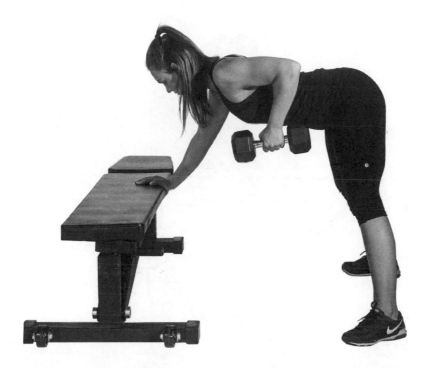

2. Draw your left shoulder blade toward the middle of your back as you simultaneously bend your elbow and row the weight to your rib cage.

3. Pause for a full second in this position. Then slowly lower the weight back down to the starting position. Complete all repetitions on the left arm before switching sides.

FORM TIP: Do not rotate your torso during the lifting phase of this exercise; keep your back and core perfectly still.

Bent-Over Dumbbell
Rear-Deltoid Raise

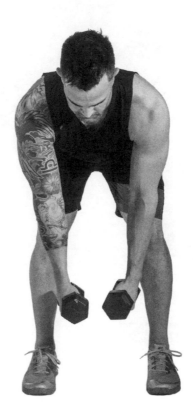

1. Stand with your feet shoulder width apart, holding a dumbbell in each hand. Push your hips back and bend over until your upper body is parallel to the floor, with your arms hanging straight down, palms facing each other and elbows straight.

WHAT IT DOES:
Strengthens the
muscles in your upper
back and rear
shoulders.

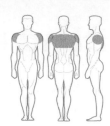

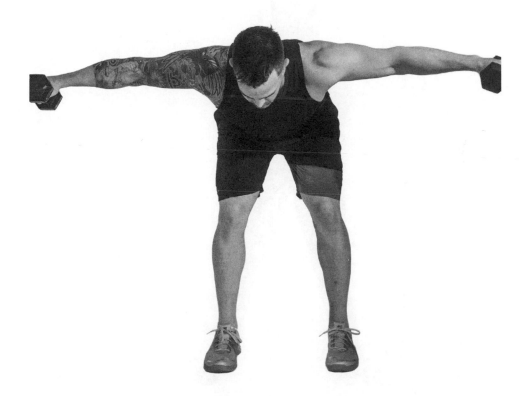

2. Using the upper-back muscles, slowly raise the dumbbells out to your sides until your arms are parallel to the floor. Make sure to keep your neck in a straight line with your back. Pause for a full second in this position before lowering the dumbbells back to the starting position, and repeat for the suggested number of reps.

FORM TIP: Use a conservative weight. Avoid using momentum to throw the dumbbells up to the sides.

Band Pull-Apart

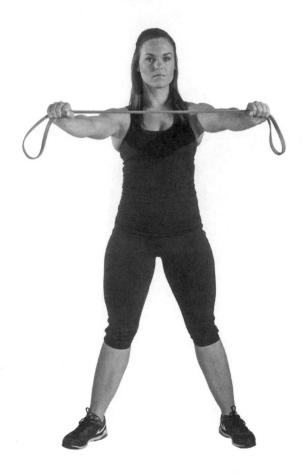

1. Stand with your feet shoulder width apart. Using an overhand grip, hold a light to moderate resistance band with your hands about shoulder width apart. Keeping your arms straight, raise them directly out in front of you.

2. Keeping your arms straight, pull the band apart until the band contacts your chest.

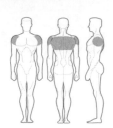

WHAT IT DOES:
Strengthens the muscles in your upper back and rear shoulders.

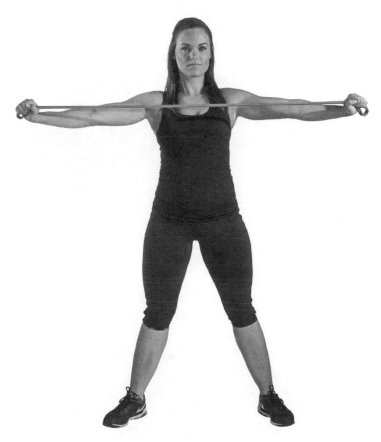

3. Pause for a full second with the band contacting your chest before returning to the starting position. Repeat for the suggested number of reps.

FORM TIP: Moving your hands out farther on the band makes this exercise easier, and moving your hands closer together on the band makes it harder. Experiment with your hand position to find the ideal tension.

Bent-Over Band Lat Pulldown

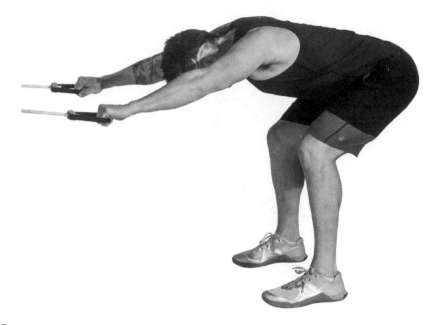

1. Anchor a moderate resistance band to a secure implement (such as a railing or a bed frame) at about chest level. Grab the handles and step back until the band develops a moderate amount of tension. Set your feet about shoulder width apart. Push your hips back and bend over until your upper body is nearly parallel to the floor. Your arms should be straight out in front of you.

WHAT IT DOES:
Strengthens the large muscles in your back that run along the sides of your spine, as well as the muscles in the front of your arms.

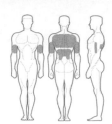

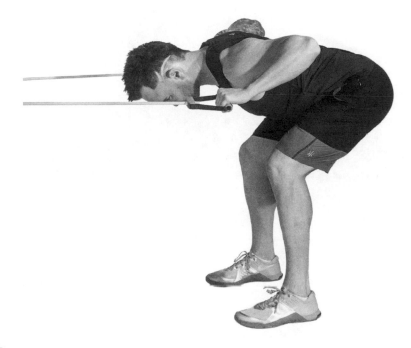

2. Pull the band handles in toward you, keeping your knuckles up and elbows out, until your hands nearly reach your shoulders.

3. Pause for a full second in this position before letting your arms back out, and repeat for the suggested number of reps.

FORM TIP: Squeeze hard from the underarms, as if you were crushing oranges in your armpits, to maximize the contraction in the target muscles.

Dumbbell Pullover

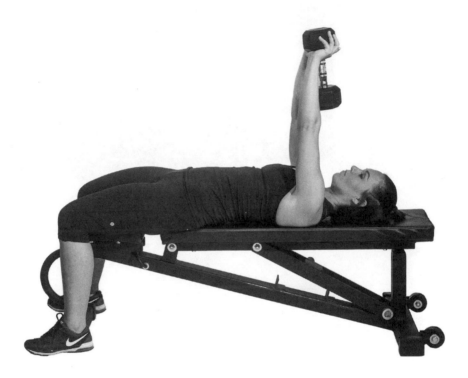

1. Lie on your back on a flat bench with your feet pressed firmly into the floor. Make a "diamond" out of your hands, with one hand on top of the other, and place the head of a dumbbell between your hands.

2. Raise your arms above your chest with the dumbbell hanging down from above. Keeping your arms straight, slowly lower the dumbbell back behind your head until you feel a comfortable stretch in your rib cage.

WHAT IT DOES:
Strengthens the large muscles in your back that run along the sides of your spine, as well as the muscles in the back of your arms and your chest.

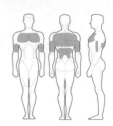

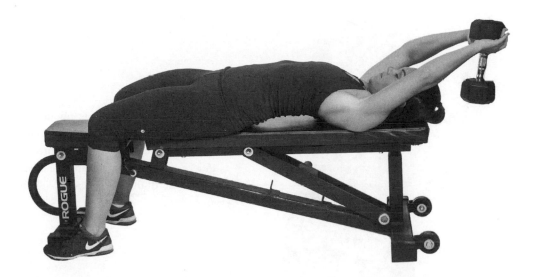

3. Once you reach this position, immediately raise the dumbbell back to the starting position, and repeat for the suggested number of reps.

FORM TIP: To engage your core and protect your lower back, push your lower back into the bench during the lowering phase of the exercise. Don't bend your elbows to lower the dumbbells; keeping your arms straight recruits the target muscles more effectively.

Dumbbell **Goblet Squat**

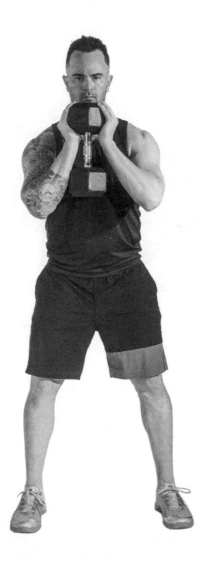

1. Stand with your feet about hip width apart. Cup one end of a dumbbell in the heels of your hands directly underneath your chin, letting the other end of the dumbbell hang and touch your chest.

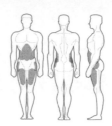

WHAT IT DOES:
Strengthens all the muscles in your hips and thighs while developing core stability.

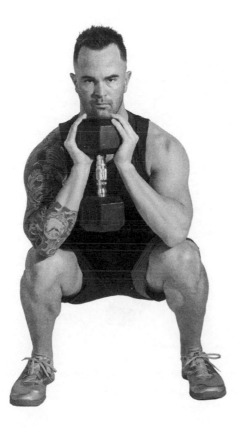

2. Tighten your abdominals and push your hips back before bending your knees and lowering yourself down into a full squat where your thighs are below parallel to the floor, as low as you can comfortably go. Be sure not to bend at the waist or come up on the balls of your feet; your weight should be back on your heels.

3. Drive back up through your heels to the starting position. Repeat for the suggested number of reps.

FORM TIP: To avoid injuring the knees, do not bounce when coming up out of the squat.

2-Stage Dumbbell
Goblet Squat

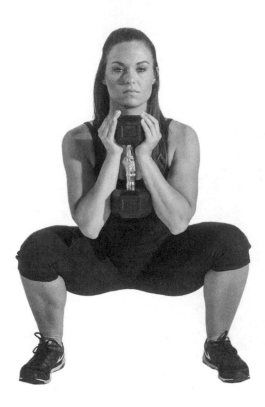

1. Stand with your feet about hip width apart. Cup one end of a dumbbell in the heels of your hands directly underneath your chin, letting the other end of the dumbbell hang and touch your chest.

2. Tighten your abdominals and push your hips back before bending your knees and lowering yourself down into a full squat where your thighs are below parallel to the floor, as low as you can comfortably go. This is the first of your 2 stages. Be sure not to bend at the waist or come up on the balls of your feet; your weight should be back on your heels.

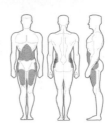

WHAT IT DOES:
Strengthens all the muscles in your hips and thighs while developing core stability.

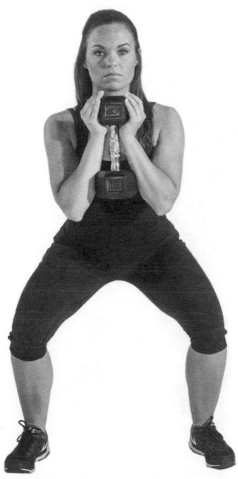

3. Stand halfway back up (the second of your 2 stages) before immediately sinking back down into the full squat position, and then immediately stand back up into the starting position. This is one full rep. Repeat for the suggested number of reps.

FORM TIP: To avoid injuring the knees, do not bounce when coming up out of the squat.

Dumbbell **Sumo Squat**

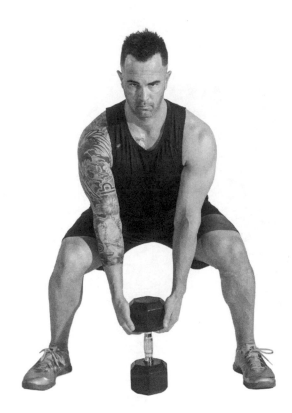

1. Place a dumbbell on the floor with one head down and one head up. Hover over the dumbbell, standing with your feet wider than hip width apart and your toes turned out to about 45 degrees. Bend your knees and lower yourself down into a squat with your fingertips cupping the head of the dumbbell. Be sure not to bend at the waist or come up on the balls of your feet; your weight should be back on your heels.

WHAT IT DOES:
Strengthens all the
muscles in your hips
and thighs.

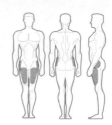

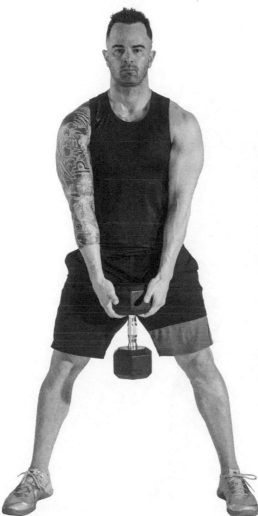

2. Drive back up through your heels to stand upright, still holding the dumbbell with your fingertips cupping its head.

3. Push your hips back and squat back down until the bottom head of the dumbbell contacts the floor. Repeat for the suggested number of reps.

FORM TIP: To avoid injuring your lower back, make sure you lead with your chest—not allowing your hips to come up first—when coming up out of the squat.

Dumbbell **Front Squat**

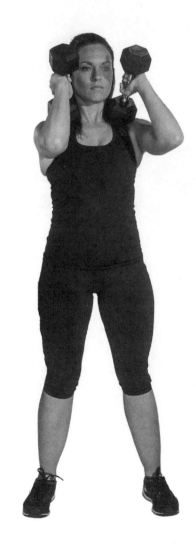

1. Stand with your feet slightly wider than shoulder width apart. Hold a dumbbell in each hand, resting the dumbbells lightly on your shoulders as if in a rack, with your elbows pointed slightly up and your palms facing in.

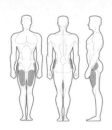

WHAT IT DOES:
Strengthens all the muscles in your hips and thighs.

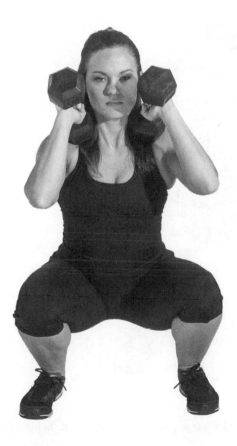

2. Bend your knees and lower yourself down into a full squat where your thighs are below parallel to the floor, as low as you can comfortably go. Be sure not to bend at the waist or come up on the balls of your feet; your weight should be back on your heels.

3. Drive back up through your heels to the starting position. Repeat for the suggested number of reps.

FORM TIP: To avoid injuring your back, keep your back straight and do not allow your elbows to dip down toward the floor.

Jump **Squat**

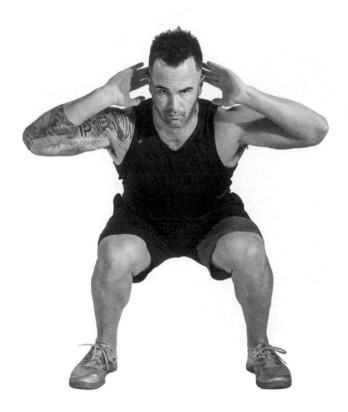

1. Stand with your feet slightly wider than shoulder width apart. Place your hands behind your head with your elbows out to the side.

2. Bend your knees and lower yourself down into a half squat with your thighs parallel to the floor. Be sure not to bend at the waist or come up on the balls of your feet; your weight should be back on your heels.

WHAT IT DOES:
Strengthens all the muscles in your hips and thighs, while developing total-body power and explosiveness.

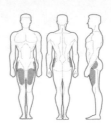

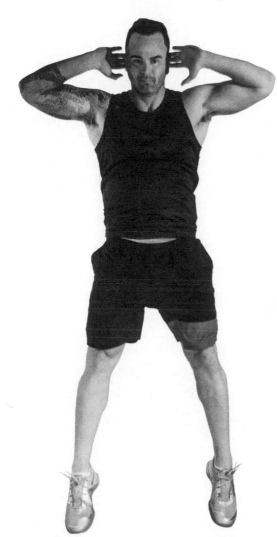

3. Drive through your heels and explode back up, jumping off the floor as high as possible.

4. As you land, keep your knees bent and immediately squat down again until your thighs are once again parallel to the floor. Repeat for the suggested number of reps.

FORM TIP: To protect your knees, avoid landing on the balls of your feet. Instead, land on your whole foot with your weight evenly distributed.

Wall **Sit**

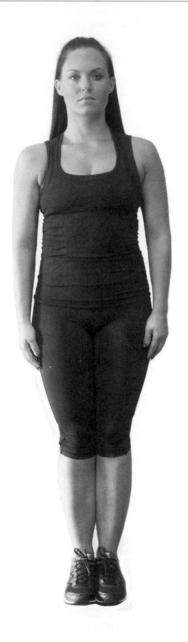

1. Stand against a wall with your head and back leaning against it.

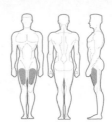

WHAT IT DOES:
Strengthens the
muscles in the front
of your thighs.

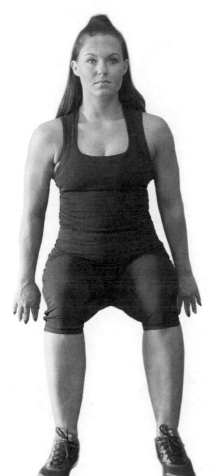

2. Slide down the wall, walking your feet out until your thighs are parallel to the floor. Hold this position for the suggested amount of time.

FORM TIP: To intensify this exercise, push your feet into the floor as though you were trying to straighten your legs.

Supported Body Weight
Split Squat

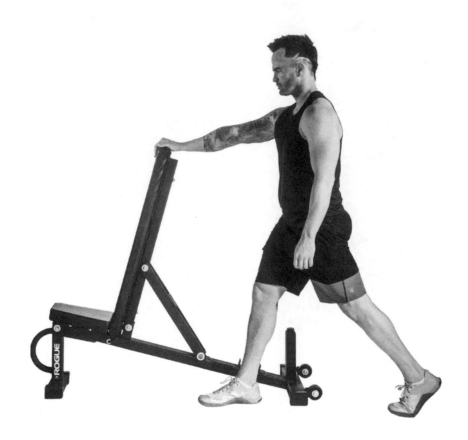

1. Holding on to a secure surface (an upright bench, a door frame, or a post) at shoulder height with your right hand, stand with your right leg forward and flat on the ground and your left leg behind, with just the ball of your left foot on the ground.

WHAT IT DOES:
Strengthens all the muscles in your hips and thighs.

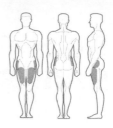

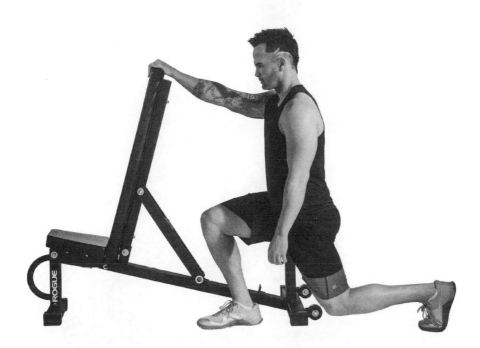

2. Bend your knees and lower yourself straight down into a half squat, where your right thigh is parallel to the floor. Keep your posture upright and your right heel on the ground.

3. Stand back up to the starting position. Repeat for the suggested number of reps before switching legs.

FORM TIP: It is important to find a comfortable stance. Do not have your legs staggered too far apart or too close together; about 2 feet between the front heel and the back toe is ideal.

Rear Foot-Elevated
Split Squat

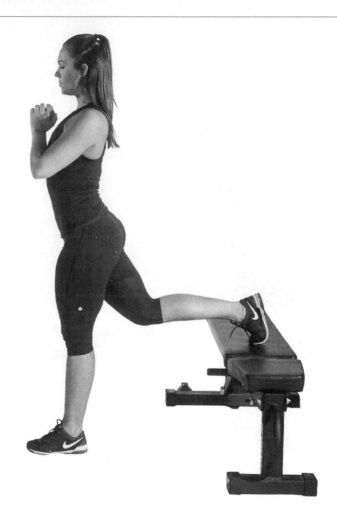

1. With your back to a flat bench, stand with your left leg forward and left foot flat on the ground and your right leg stretched behind you with the ball of your right foot on the bench.

WHAT IT DOES:
Strengthens the
muscles in the front
of your thighs.

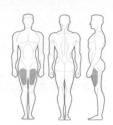

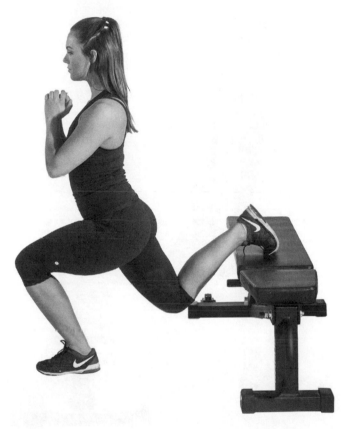

2. Bend your knees and lower yourself down into a half squat where your left thigh is parallel to the floor. Keep your posture upright and your weight on your left heel.

3. Drive through your left heel to stand back up to the starting position. Repeat for the suggested number of reps before switching legs.

FORM TIP: If you have trouble balancing during this exercise, hold on to a support about chest height (the frame of a squat rack, a bed frame, or a railing).

Rear Foot-Elevated
Isometric Split Squat

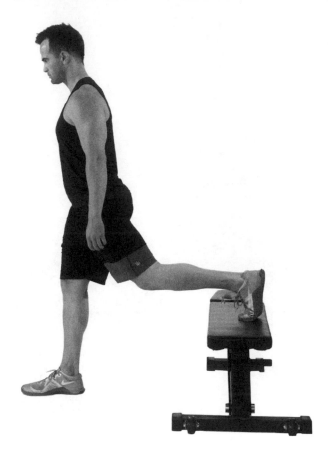

1. With your back to a flat bench, stand with your right leg forward and right foot flat on the ground and your left leg stretched behind you with the ball of your left foot on the bench.

2. Bend your knees and lower yourself down into a half squat where your right thigh is parallel to the floor. Keep your posture upright and your weight on your right heel.

WHAT IT DOES:
Strengthens all the
muscles in your hips
and thighs.

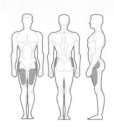

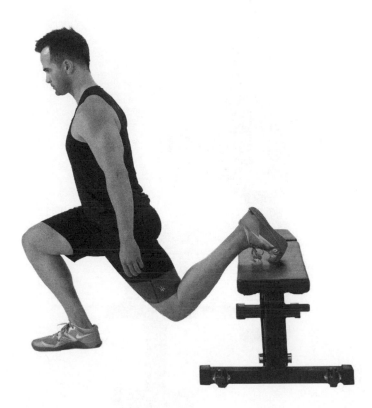

3. Hold for the suggested amount of time.

4. Drive through your right heel to stand back up to the starting position. Switch legs and repeat for the suggested amount of time.

FORM TIP: To enhance your balance during this exercise, drive hard through the heel of your working leg.

Dumbbell **Step-Up**

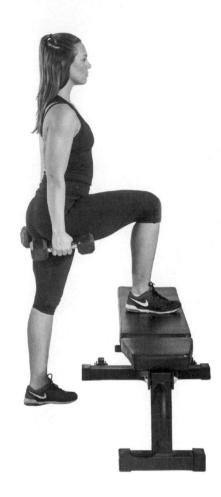

1. Stand facing a flat bench with your feet together, holding a dumbbell in each hand with your arms hanging down at your sides. Place your right foot on the bench with your right knee at a 90-degree angle. Your left leg should be directly under your hips, and your left foot should be flat on the floor. Keep an upright posture with your shoulder blades pulled back.

WHAT IT DOES:
Strengthens all the muscles in your hips and thighs.

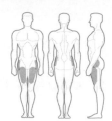

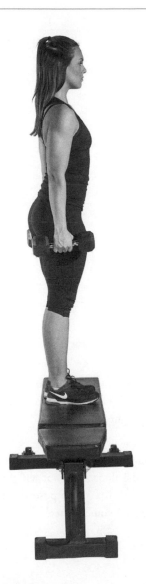

2. Drive through your right heel to step up and onto the bench with your left foot, straightening both legs.

3. Pause for a full second in the upright position. Slowly lower your left leg back down to the floor. Repeat for the suggested number of reps before switching legs.

FORM TIP: When you step up and onto the bench, avoid propelling yourself off the floor with your rear leg. Instead, focus on using the leg that is up on the bench.

Alternating Body Weight
Reverse Lunge

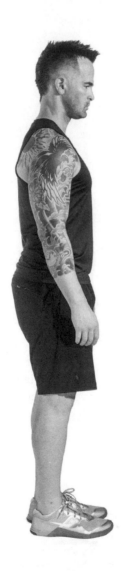

1. Stand with your feet together.

2. Keeping your left foot planted, lunge your right leg back behind you, moving onto the ball of your right foot.

3. Squat straight down until your right knee nearly reaches the floor and your left thigh is parallel to the floor. Keep your posture upright and your weight on your left heel.

WHAT IT DOES:
Strengthens all the muscles in your hips and thighs.

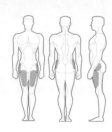

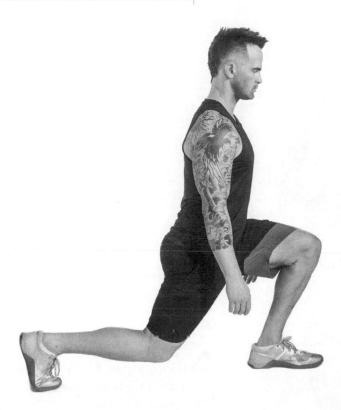

4. Stand back up and into the starting position. Switch legs, lunging back with your left leg. Repeat, in alternating fashion, for the suggested number of reps on each side.

FORM TIP: Don't lunge too far back. If you are having trouble keeping your balance or are feeling an extreme stretch in your rear leg, you are over-striding and should move your feet a little closer together.

Alternating Goblet
Reverse Lunge

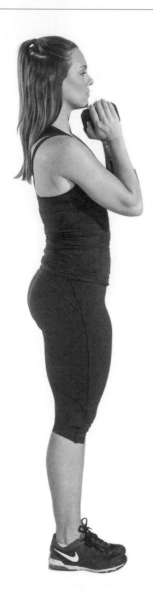

1. Stand with your feet about hip width apart. Cup one end of a dumbbell in the heels of your hands directly underneath your chin, with the other end of the dumbbell touching your chest.

2. Keeping your left foot planted, lunge your right leg behind you, moving onto the ball of your right foot.

3. Squat straight down until your right knee nearly reaches the floor and your left thigh is parallel to the floor. Keep your posture upright and your weight on your left heel.

WHAT IT DOES:
Strengthens all the
muscles in your hips
and thighs.

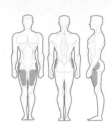

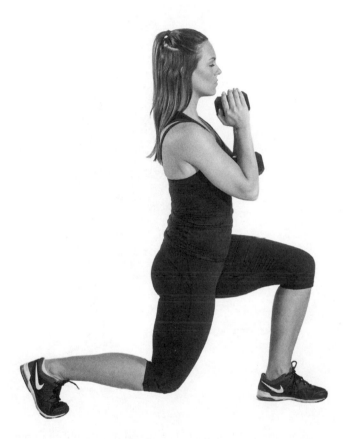

4. Stand back up to the starting position. Switch legs, lunging back with your left leg. Repeat, in alternating fashion, for the suggested number of reps on each side.

FORM TIP: Don't lunge too far back. If you are having trouble keeping your balance or are feeling an extreme stretch in the rear leg, you are overstriding and should move your feet closer together.

Goblet Combination **Lunge**

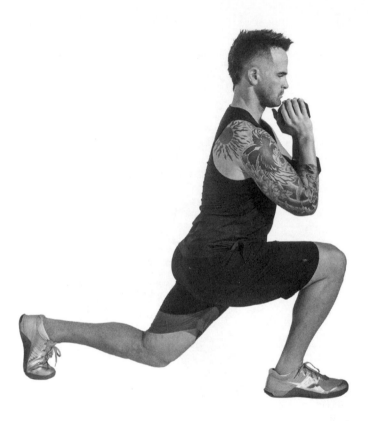

1. Stand with your feet about hip width apart. Cup one end of a dumbbell in the heels of your hands directly underneath your chin, with the other end of the dumbbell touching your chest.

2. Keeping your right foot planted, lunge your left leg back behind you, moving onto the ball of your left foot. Squat straight down until your left knee nearly reaches the floor and your right thigh is parallel to the floor. Keep your posture upright and your weight on your right heel.

3. Stand back up to the starting position.

WHAT IT DOES:
Strengthens all the
muscles in your hips
and thighs.

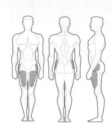

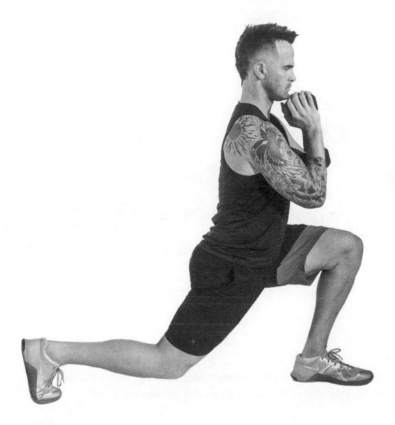

4. Keeping the ball of your right foot planted, lunge forward with the left leg until the left thigh is parallel to the floor and your right knee nearly touches the floor.

5. Propel yourself back to the starting position by pushing through your left foot. Lunge back and forth with your left foot for the suggested number of reps before switching sides.

FORM TIP: To avoid losing balance, pause for a full second in the upright position before transitioning to the other direction.

Stability Ball **Hip Extension**

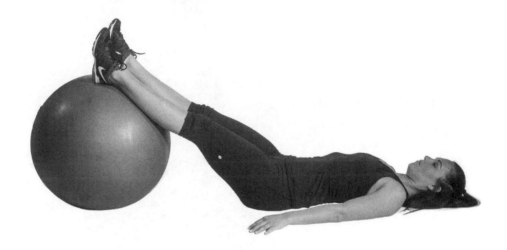

1. Lie on your back with your legs straight and elevated onto a stability ball just below your calves. Your hands should be flat on the floor with your palms down.

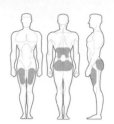

WHAT IT DOES:
Strengthens the muscles
in the back of your thighs,
your rear end, and your
lower back.

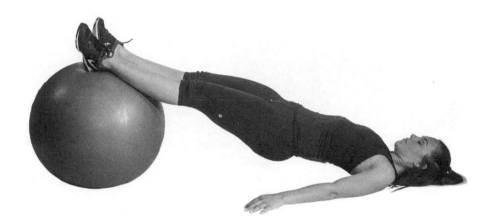

2. Keeping your abdominals tight, press your lower legs into the ball and push your hips into the air until they are level with your back, forming a bridge.

3. Pause in this position for a full second. Slowly lower your hips back down to the ground. Repeat for the suggested number of reps.

FORM TIP: When you are in the bridge position, really squeeze your rear end.

Single-Leg **Glute Bridge**

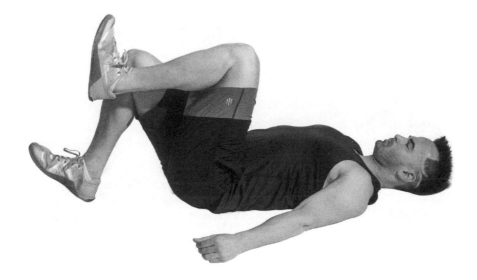

1. Lie on your back with your knees bent at a 90-degree angle and both feet on the floor. Flex your left hip, pick your left foot up, and bend your left knee back until it is over your waist.

WHAT IT DOES:
Strengthens the muscles
in the back of your thighs,
your rear end, and your
lower back.

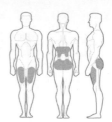

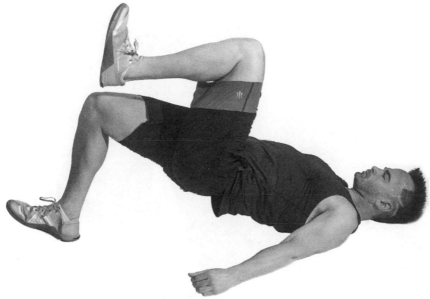

2. Drive your right heel into the floor and push your hips up and into the air to form a bridge. Your knees, hips, and shoulders should form a straight line. You should feel a strong contraction in your right butt cheek.

3. Pause for a full second in this position. Slowly lower your hips back to the ground. Repeat for the suggested number of reps before switching sides.

FORM TIP: When you are in the bridge position, really squeeze your rear end.

Hip **Thrust**

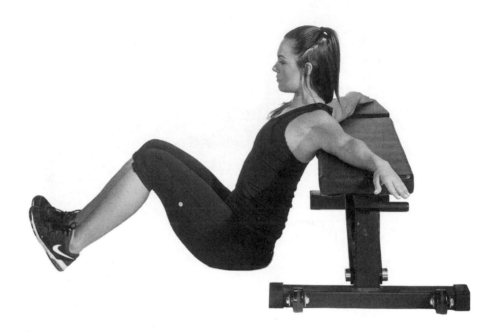

1. Sit on the floor with your upper back resting against a flat bench just below your shoulder blades. Your arms should be straight out to the sides resting on the bench with your palms facing down on the bench. Your legs should be bent at a 90-degree angle with your ankles flexed (pull your toes to your shins).

WHAT IT DOES:
Strengthens the muscles in the back of your thighs, your rear end, and your lower back.

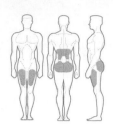

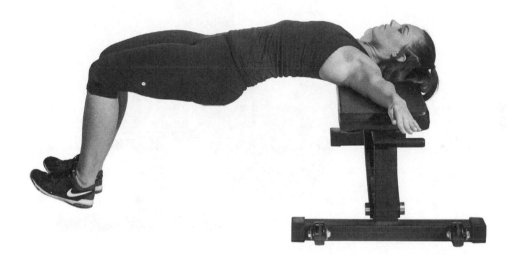

2. Drive your heels through the floor and push your hips up and into the air until they are parallel to the floor, forming a bridge.

3. Pause for a full second in this position. Slowly lower your hips back down to the floor. Repeat for the suggested number of reps.

FORM TIP: To intensify the contraction in your rear end, when you are in the bridge position, tilt your pelvis back, rolling your hip bones back toward your rib cage.

Single-Leg **Hip Thrust**

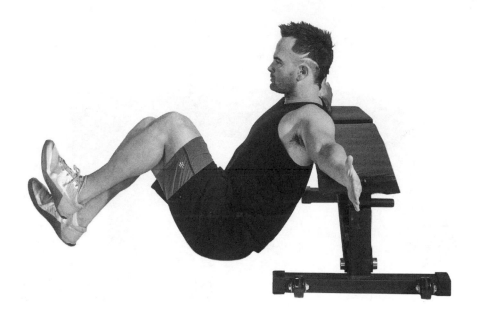

1. Sit on the floor with your upper back resting against a flat bench just below your shoulder blades. Your arms should be straight out to the sides with your palms facing forward. Both of your legs should be bent at a 90-degree angle with your ankles flexed (pull your toes to your shins). Flex your left hip slightly, so that your left knee comes slightly back toward your chest and your left foot comes off the ground.

WHAT IT DOES:
Strengthens the muscles
in the back of your thighs,
your rear end, and your
lower back.

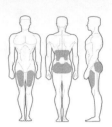

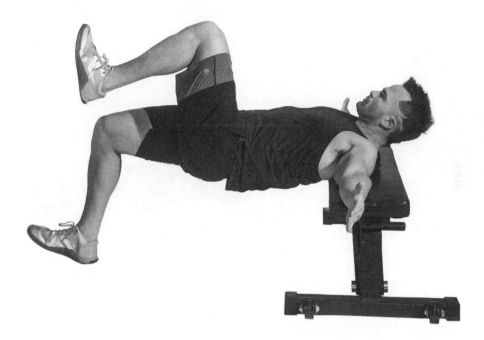

3. Using your right leg, drive through your right heel and push your hips up and into the air until your back and hips are parallel to the floor, forming a bridge. Your left knee should stay pulled slightly back toward your chest.

4. Pause for a full second in this position. Slowly lower your hips back down to the floor. Repeat for the suggested number of reps before switching legs.

FORM TIP: To avoid straining your neck, don't allow your head to sag behind you.

Stability Ball **Leg Curl**

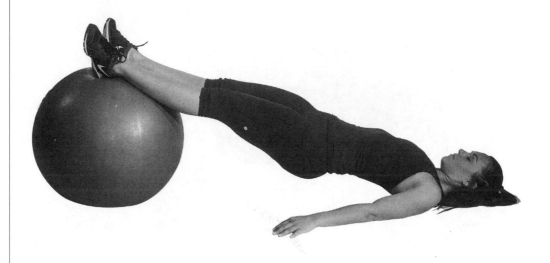

1. Lie on your back with your legs straight and elevated onto a stability ball just below your calves. Your hands should be flat on the floor with the palms down.

2. Tighten your abdominals, press your lower legs into the ball, and push your hips up and into the air. Your knees, hips, and shoulders should form a straight line.

WHAT IT DOES:
Strengthens the muscles in the back of your thighs, your rear end, and your lower back.

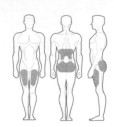

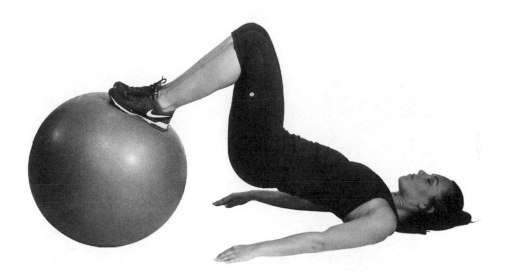

3. Bend your knees and pull your heels as far as you can toward your rear end.

4. Extend your legs back out and lower your hips back down to the floor to the starting position. Repeat for the suggested number of reps.

FORM TIP: To avoid losing balance, do not rush. Instead, break this exercise into parts: up, in, out, down.

Dumbbell **Romanian Deadlift**

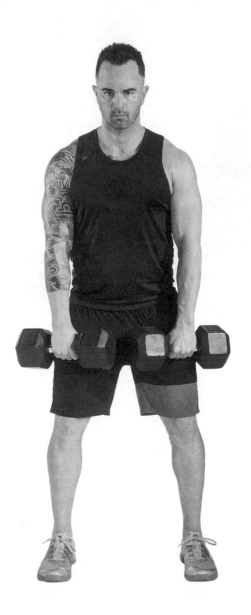

1. Stand with your feet shoulder width apart, holding a dumbbell in each hand hanging at arm's length, with your hands on the front of your thighs.

WHAT IT DOES:
Strengthens the muscles in the back of your thighs, your rear end, and your lower back.

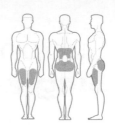

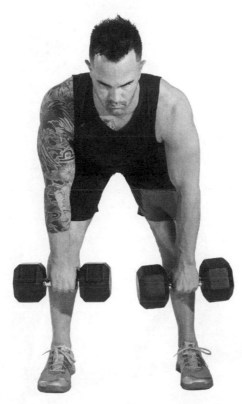

2. Slowly push your hips back and lean forward, allowing the dumbbells to travel directly down your legs until they reach the middle of your shins. You should feel a mild stretch in the back of your thighs.

3. Extend back up to the starting position. Repeat for the suggested number of reps.

FORM TIP: To avoid injuring your lower back, do not bend over at the waist. Your back should remain perfectly flat.

Supported Body Weight
Single-Leg Romanian Deadlift

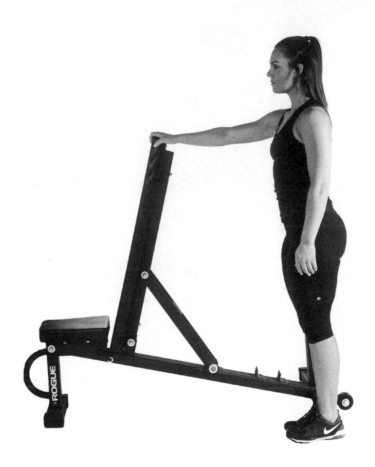

1. Stand with your feet together, holding a secure surface (an upright bench, a door frame, or a post) with your right hand at about shoulder level.

WHAT IT DOES:
Strengthens the muscles in the back of your thighs, your rear end, and your lower back.

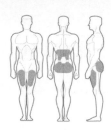

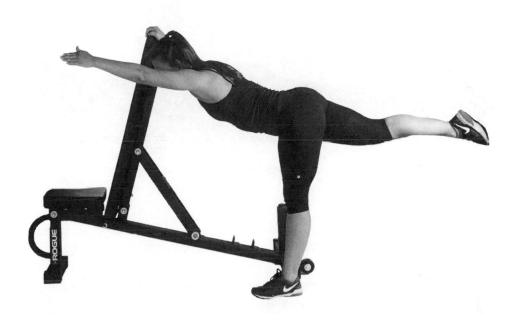

2. Lift your right foot off the floor a couple of inches. Push back through your left hip and lean forward until your upper body becomes parallel with the ground. Allow your right leg to trail behind you and your left arm to move out in front of you.

3. Once you feel a mild stretch in the back of your left thigh, extend back up to the starting position and pause for a full second to check your form. Perform the suggested number of reps before switching sides.

FORM TIP: To avoid injuring your lower back, do not bend over at the waist. Your back should remain perfectly flat.

Prone **Cobra**

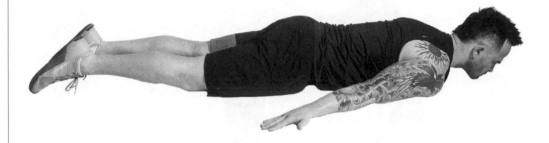

1. Lie facedown with your legs together, chin resting on the floor, and your arms alongside your upper body with your palms flat on the ground.

2. Squeeze your rear end and slowly lift your head, chest, and arms off the floor while simultaneously squeezing your shoulder blades together.

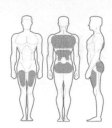

WHAT IT DOES:
Strengthens the muscles in the back of your thighs, your rear end, and your upper and lower back.

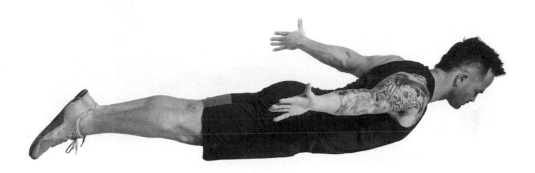

3. Pause for a full second in this position. Lower your head and chest back down to the floor. Repeat for the suggested number of reps.

FORM TIP: To avoid hyperextending your lower back, don't lift up too far. You need to lift up only a few inches. You should feel this exercise primarily in your rear end and upper-back muscles.

Plank

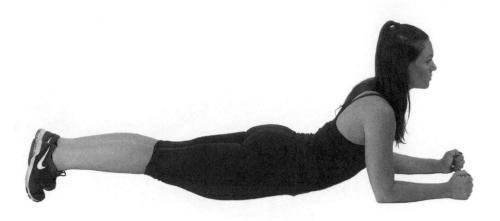

1. Assume a plank position, resting on your elbows, with the balls of your feet about shoulder width apart. Your elbows should be directly underneath your shoulders, your back should be flat, and your neck should form a straight line with your back. Tighten your rear end and abdominals and the front of the thighs.

WHAT IT DOES:
Strengthens
the entire core.

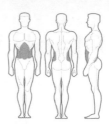

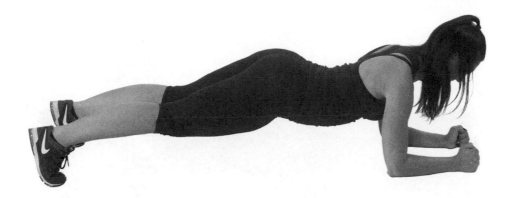

2. Hold this position for the suggested amount of time. Do not allow your lower back to sag.

FORM TIP: To intensify this exercise, narrow your base of support by moving your feet closer together.

Plank **Walk-Up**

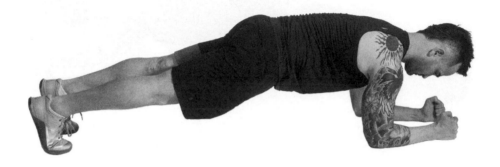

1. Assume a plank position, resting on your elbows, with the balls of your feet about shoulder width apart. Your elbows should be directly underneath your shoulders, your back should be flat, and your neck should form a straight line with your back. Tighten your rear end, abdominals, and the front of the thighs.

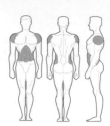

WHAT IT DOES:
Strengthens the entire core and increases shoulder strength and stability.

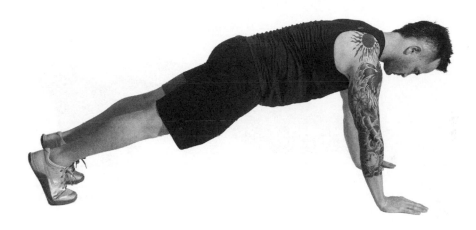

2. Plant your right hand on the ground and push up, then do the same with your left hand, to walk up and onto your hands.

3. Reverse the movement going back down, moving onto one elbow at a time. Repeat for the suggested number of reps, not allowing your lower back to sag.

FORM TIP: To intensify this exercise, bring your feet together and narrow your base of support.

Long Lever **Plank**

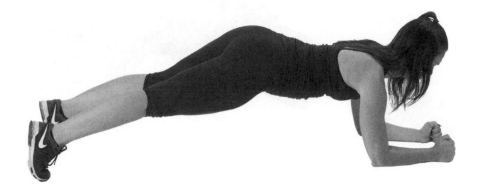

1. Assume a plank position, resting on your elbows, with the balls of your feet about shoulder width apart. Your elbows should be a few inches in front of your shoulders, forming a longer lever than in a standard plank. Your back should be flat, and your neck should form a straight line with your back. Tighten your rear end, abdominals, and the front of the thighs.

WHAT IT DOES:
Strengthens the
entire core.

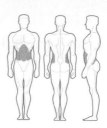

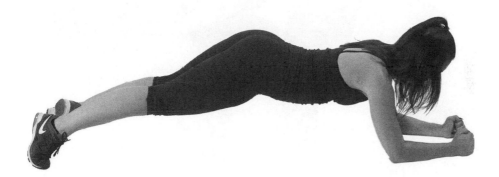

2. Hold this position for the suggested amount of time, not allowing your lower back to sag.

FORM TIP: To intensify this exercise, bring your feet together and narrow your base of support.

Inch **Worm**

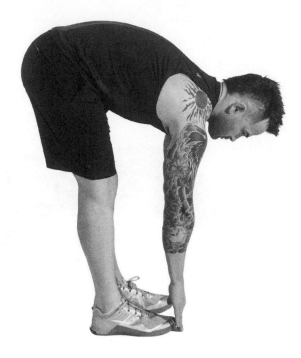

1. Stand with your feet together. Bend at your waist and touch your toes. Keep your knees as straight as possible, but if you need to bend them to reach your toes, go ahead and do so.

WHAT IT DOES:
Strengthens your entire core, increases shoulder stability, and stretches and lengthens the back of your thighs.

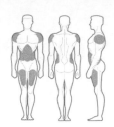

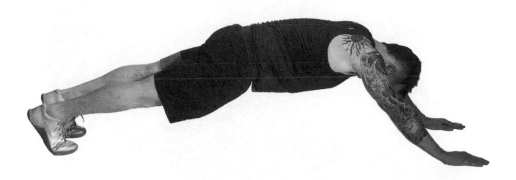

2. Slowly walk your hands away from your feet, inching your way forward until your body is parallel, or near parallel, to the floor and your hands are about a foot in front of your shoulders. Pause for a full second in this position.

3. Keeping your abdominals and rear end tight and your back flat, walk your way slowly back into the starting position and repeat for the suggested number of reps.

FORM TIP: Do not move through this movement too fast. Take your time walking in and out, and focus on tightening up your core.

Side **Plank**

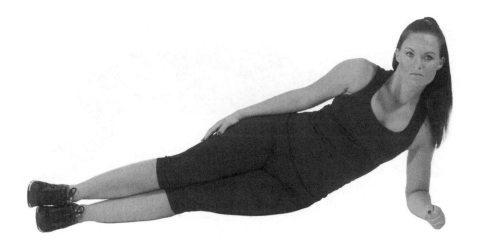

1. Lie on your left side with your left elbow propped up directly underneath your shoulder. Your legs should be straight and stacked on top of each other.

WHAT IT DOES:
Strengthens the entire core with an emphasis on the side abdominals.

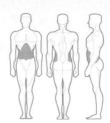

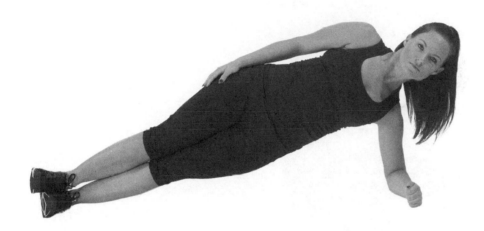

2. Tightening your abs and the front of your thighs, lift your hips up and into the air. Your body should form a straight line.

3. Hold this position, not allowing your hips to sag, for the suggested amount of time before switching sides.

FORM TIP: Make sure your top shoulder does not rotate forward, as this makes the exercise less effective for your side abdominals.

Single-Arm **Dumbbell Carry**

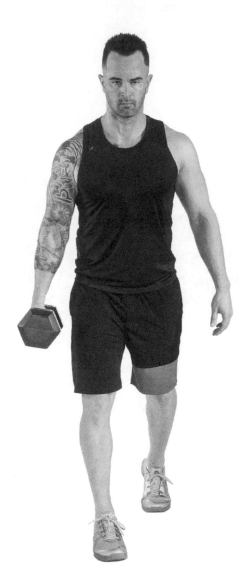

1. Stand, holding a dumbbell in your right hand, with your right arm hanging down by your body.

WHAT IT DOES:
Strengthens the entire core, with an emphasis on the side abdominals and the gripping muscles in your hands.

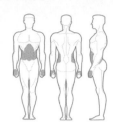

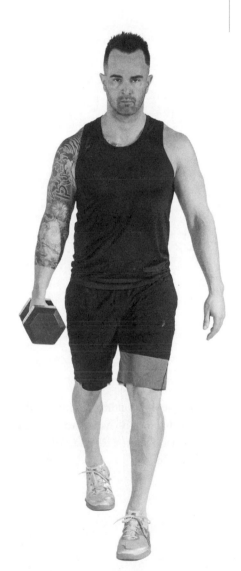

2. Keeping your right shoulder blade pulled back and the dumbbell a few inches off the side of your thigh, walk for the suggested number of steps before switching hands.

FORM TIP: Do not allow the dumbbell to pull you to the side.

Double-Arm **Dumbbell Carry**

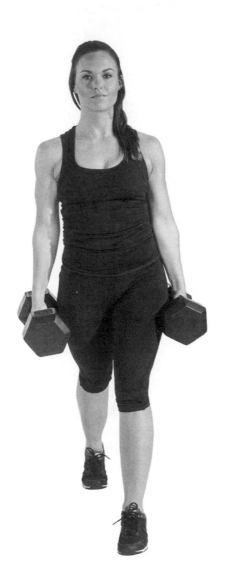

1. Stand, holding a dumbbell in each hand, with your arms hanging down by your sides and your palms facing in.

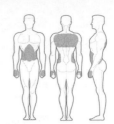

WHAT IT DOES:
Strengthens the entire
core, upper back,
and gripping muscles
in your hands.

2. Keeping your shoulders pulled back, walk at a steady pace for the suggested number of steps.

FORM TIP: To enhance the effectiveness of the exercise and the involvement of your upper back muscles, walk tall and don't allow your shoulders to hunch or round forward.

Overhead **Dumbbell Carry**

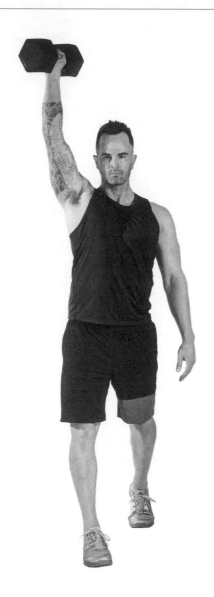

1. Stand, holding a dumbbell in your right hand over your head, with the palm facing in toward your body. Your right shoulder should be packed down into its socket.

WHAT IT DOES:
Strengthens the entire core, with an emphasis on the side abdominals, and builds shoulder stability.

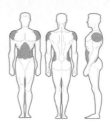

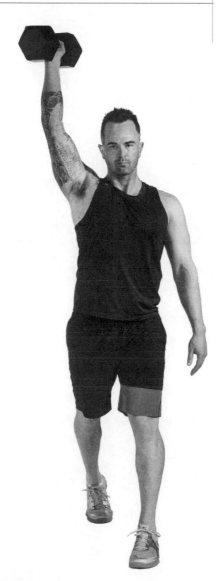

2. Keeping your right wrist straight and tightening your abdominals, walk at a steady pace for the suggested number of steps before switching arms.

FORM TIP: To avoid potential injury to the shoulder, start with a very conservative weight—20 to 30 pounds for most people—until you get the feel of the exercise.

Hollow **Body Hold**

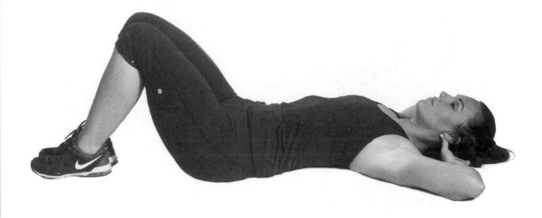

1. Lie flat on your back with your knees bent. Place your fingertips behind your ears with your elbows out.

2. Straighten your legs and raise them about a foot off the ground, keeping your lower back pressed into the floor.

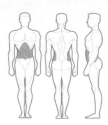

WHAT IT DOES:
Strengthens the
entire core.

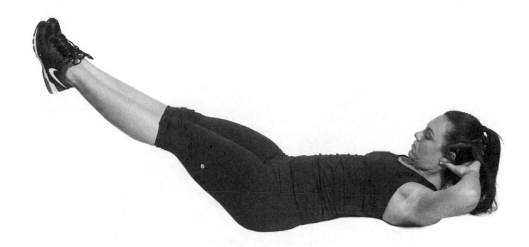

3. Slowly raise your head and shoulders off the floor.

4. Hold this position for the suggested amount of time.

FORM TIP: If the exercise is too difficult, place your hands across your chest as you crunch up and hold.

Reverse **Crunch**

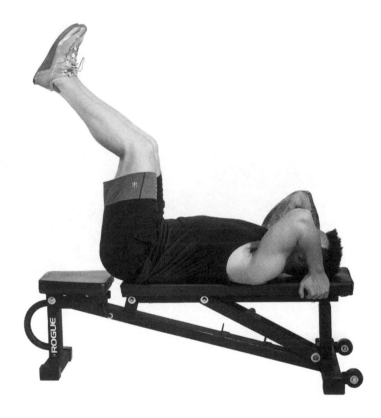

1. Lie flat on your back on a flat bench with your hands gripping the bench by your ears and your legs bent to a 90-degree angle at the knee. Bring your knees over your waist.

2. Using your lower abdomen, roll your hips back toward your rib cage until your lower back rolls off the bench a few inches and your knees come over your chest. You should not feel pressure in your neck; if you do, you've rolled too far back.

WHAT IT DOES:
Strengthens the lower abdominals.

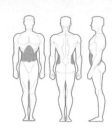

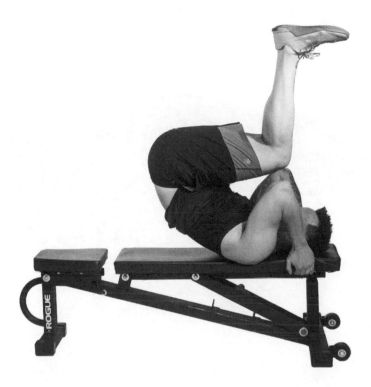

3. Reverse the motion, rolling back to the starting position where your lower back is flat against the bench. Repeat for the suggested number of reps.

FORM TIP: To avoid lower-back discomfort, do not allow your feet to come all the way back down to the bench during the lowering phase of the exercise.

Stability Ball **Crunch**

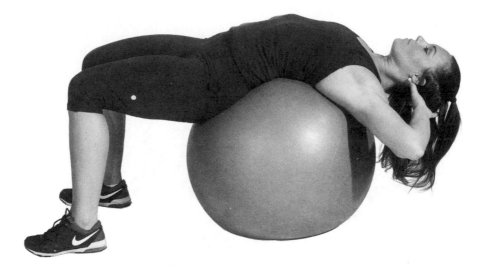

1. Lie with your lower back on top of a stability ball and your feet flat on the floor. Place your hands behind your head, your fingertips behind your ears, and your elbows out to the side.

WHAT IT DOES:
Strengthens the front and
lower abdominals.

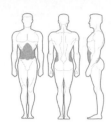

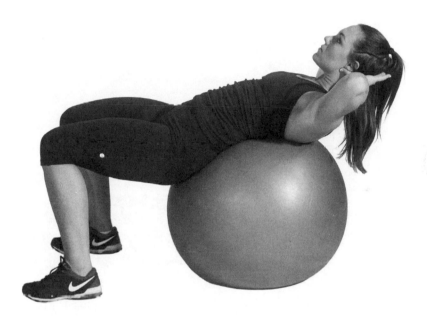

2. Lean back over the ball until you feel a stretch in your abdominals.

3. Lift your chest, head, and back until you feel a strong contraction in your abdominals. Repeat for the suggested number of reps.

FORM TIP: Don't extend so far that you fall off the back of the ball. If the exercise is too difficult, place your hands across your chest instead.

1 Back/1 Out **Crunch**

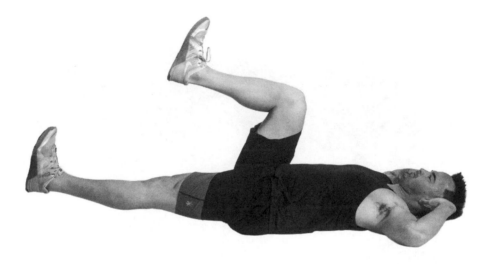

1. Lie flat on your back on the floor, with your hands behind your head, your fingertips behind your ears, and your elbows out to the side. Your right leg should be straight on the floor. Bend your left knee and lift it over your left hip. Raise your right leg straight up off the floor a few inches.

WHAT IT DOES:
Strengthens the front and
lower abdominals.

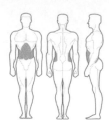

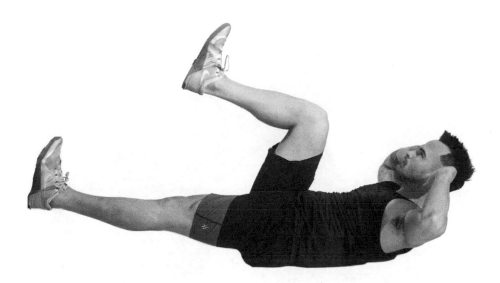

2. Lift your chest, head, and back a few inches off the floor until you feel a strong contraction in your abdominals. Repeat for the suggested number of reps before switching sides.

FORM TIP: If the exercise is too difficult, place your hands across your chest as you crunch up.

Stability Ball **Rollout**

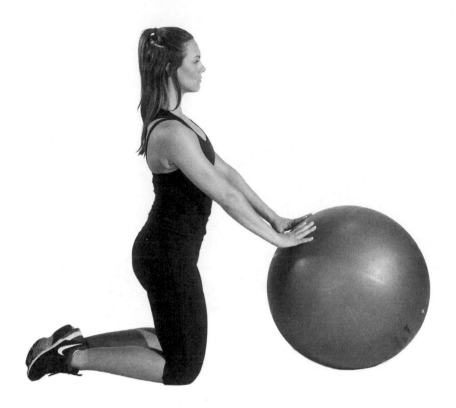

1. Kneeling in front of a stability ball, extend your arms and place your hands on the front of the ball near the top.

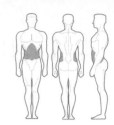

WHAT IT DOES:
Strengthens the
entire core.

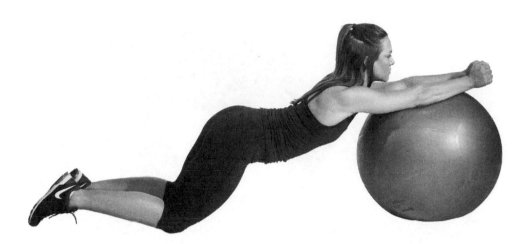

2. Keeping your back flat, tighten your abdominals and rear end and slowly roll the ball forward, allowing your forearms to go on the top of the ball. Roll out until a straight line is formed between the hips and the shoulders.

3. Pause for a full second in this position. Roll the ball back in and repeat for the suggested number of reps.

FORM TIP: Do not allow your hips to sag. If you feel discomfort in your lower back, do not roll out as far.

Stability Ball **Saw**

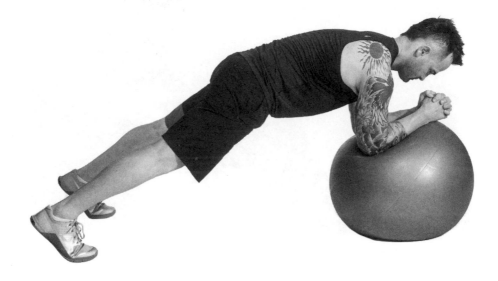

1. Assume a plank position with your elbows and forearms on an exercise ball and your feet on the floor about hip width apart.

WHAT IT DOES:
Strengthens the
entire core.

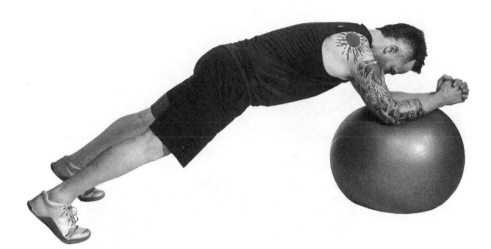

2. Keeping your back flat and your abdominals tight, slowly "saw" your elbows out just a few inches, not allowing your hips or lower back to sag.

3. Saw the elbows back in to the starting position and repeat, sawing in and out, for the suggested number of reps.

FORM TIP: Do not saw too far out; stop as soon as you feel any discomfort in your lower back.

Dying **Bug**

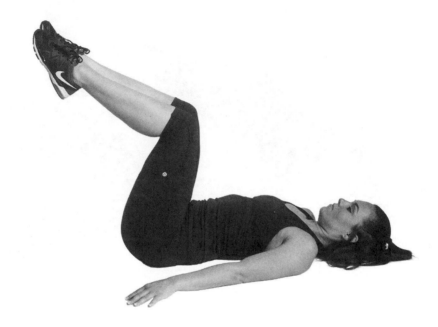

1. Lie flat on your back on the floor with both your knees over your waist and bent to a 90-degree angle. Your arms should be along the sides of the body, flat on the floor, with the palms down.

2. Keeping your lower back pressed down into the floor, slowly extend your left leg forward and down until your knee is straight.

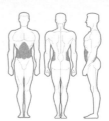

WHAT IT DOES:
Strengthens the
entire core.

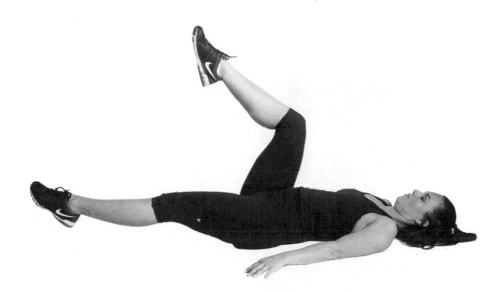

3. Pause for a full second in this position. Bend the left knee and bring the left leg back to the starting position.

4. Switch legs. Alternate, extending your left leg and then your right leg, for the suggested number of reps on each side.

FORM TIP: Prior to each rep, breathe deeply, filling your belly with air by expanding the abdominals outward.

Band Core **Press**

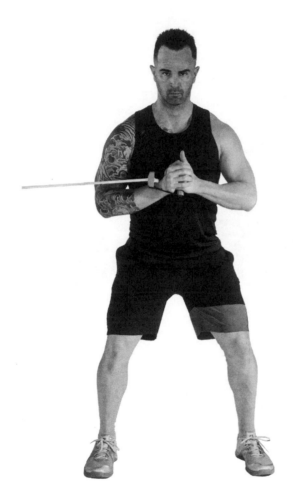

1. Anchor a resistance band to a secure surface (such as a railing or a bedpost) at about chest level. Grasp the band handle with both hands and step back until the band develops a moderate amount of tension. Stand with your feet hip width apart, squatting down slightly. Hold the band handle against your chest with your fingers interlocked and palms facing each other.

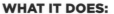

WHAT IT DOES:
Strengthens the entire core, with an emphasis on the oblique muscles that rotate your torso.

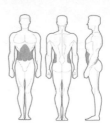

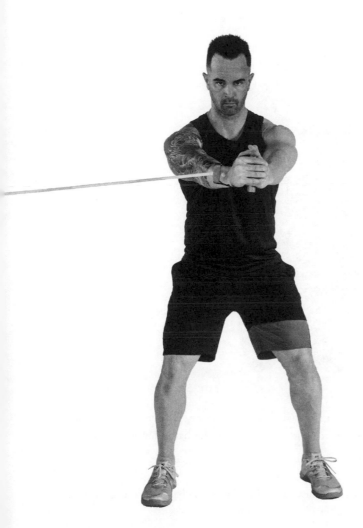

2. Tightening your rear end and abdominals, press the band out in front of you until both arms are fully extended.

3. Pause for a full second with the arms extended, not allowing the band to rotate your body. Bring the band handle back in to your chest and repeat for the suggested number of reps. Turn around and repeat on the opposite side.

FORM TIP: Do not let your hips shift or sway.

Tall Kneeling **Band Core Press**

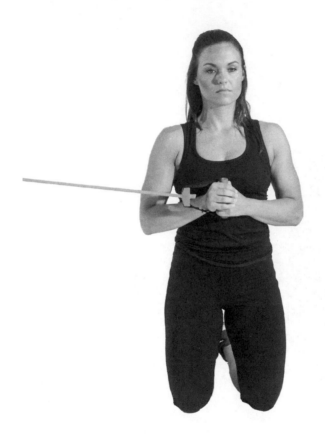

1. Anchor a resistance band to a secure surface (such as a railing or a bedpost) at about waist level. Grasp the band handle with both hands and step out until the band develops a moderate amount of tension.

2. Kneel on both knees with your knees almost touching. Hold the band handle against your chest with your fingers interlocked and palms facing each other.

WHAT IT DOES:
Strengthens the entire core, with an emphasis on the oblique muscles that rotate your torso.

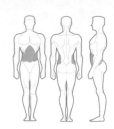

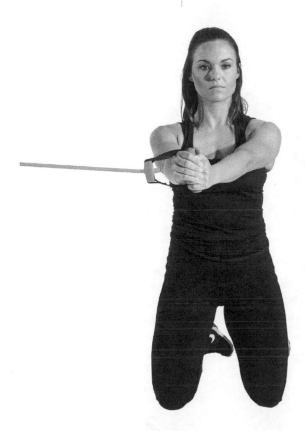

3. Tightening your rear end and abdominals, press the band out in front of you until both arms are fully extended.

4. Pause for a full second with the arms extended, not allowing the band to rotate your body. Bring the band handle back in to your chest and repeat for the suggested number of reps. Turn around and repeat on the opposite side.

FORM TIP: To really work your core muscles, avoid letting your hips shift or sway.

High-to-Low **Band Chop**

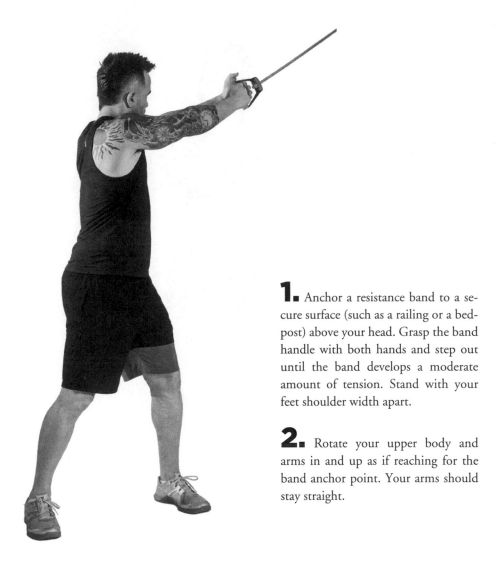

1. Anchor a resistance band to a secure surface (such as a railing or a bedpost) above your head. Grasp the band handle with both hands and step out until the band develops a moderate amount of tension. Stand with your feet shoulder width apart.

2. Rotate your upper body and arms in and up as if reaching for the band anchor point. Your arms should stay straight.

WHAT IT DOES:
Strengthens the entire core, with an emphasis on the oblique muscles that rotate your torso.

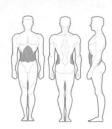

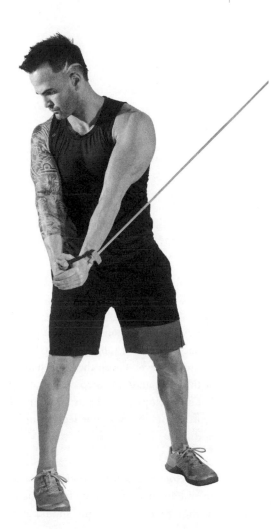

3. Using only the muscles in your core, rotate from the anchor point, through the midline of your body, and down to a point where your hands reach the outside of your right hip.

4. Pause for a full second and return to the starting position. Repeat for the suggested number of reps, turn around, and repeat on the other side.

FORM TIP: Perform this movement smoothly and slowly, and avoid pulling too hard with your arms; think of them solely as a connector to the band handles.

Low-to-High **Band Chop**

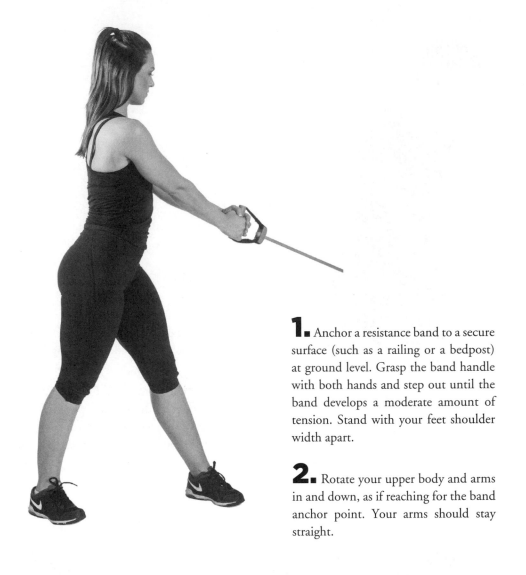

1. Anchor a resistance band to a secure surface (such as a railing or a bedpost) at ground level. Grasp the band handle with both hands and step out until the band develops a moderate amount of tension. Stand with your feet shoulder width apart.

2. Rotate your upper body and arms in and down, as if reaching for the band anchor point. Your arms should stay straight.

WHAT IT DOES:
Strengthens the entire core, with an emphasis on the oblique muscles that rotate your torso.

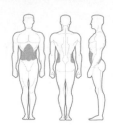

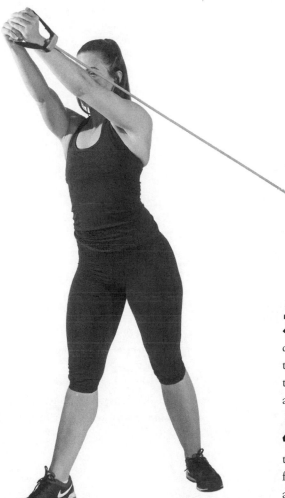

3. Using only the muscles in your core, rotate from the low position, through the midline of your body, and to a point where your hands are up above your left shoulder.

4. Pause for a full second and return to the starting position. Repeat for the suggested number of reps, turn around, and repeat on the other side.

FORM TIP: Perform this movement smoothly and slowly, and avoid pulling too hard with your arms; think of them solely as a connector to the band handles.

Run in **Place**

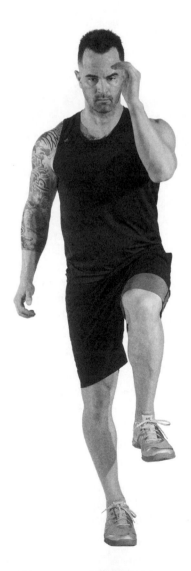

1. Stand with your feet together.

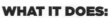

WHAT IT DOES:
Develops cardiovascular conditioning.

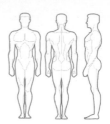

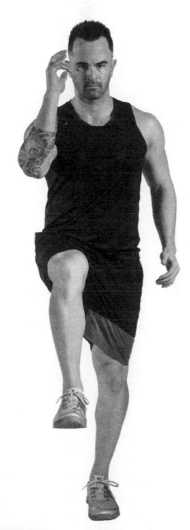

2. Tightening your abdominals, vigorously run in place, lifting your knees as high as you can and pumping your arms back and forth. Continue for the suggested amount of time.

FORM TIP: Be as light on your feet as possible and drive your arms and legs in a piston-like motion.

Phantom **Rope Skipping**

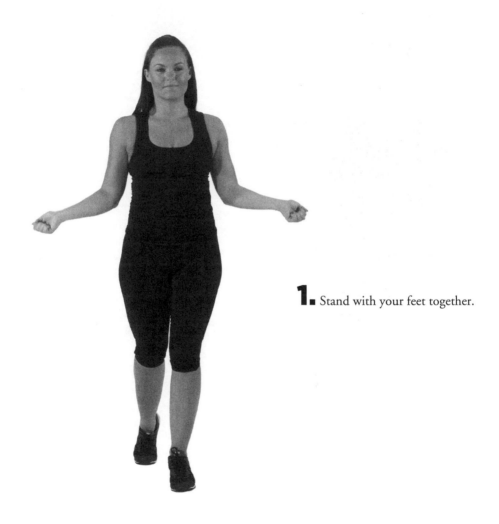

1. Stand with your feet together.

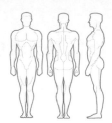

WHAT IT DOES:
Develops cardiovascular conditioning.

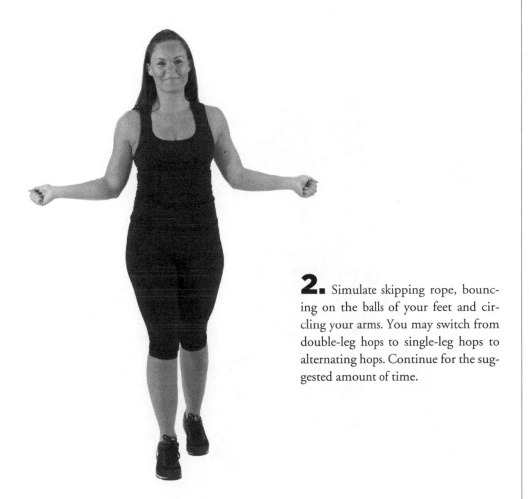

2. Simulate skipping rope, bouncing on the balls of your feet and circling your arms. You may switch from double-leg hops to single-leg hops to alternating hops. Continue for the suggested amount of time.

FORM TIP: Be as light on your feet as possible and develop a rhythm.

Side-to-Side **Shuffle**

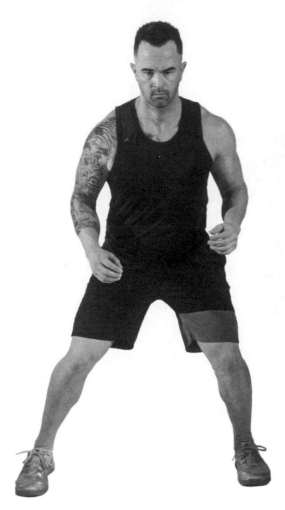

1. Stand with your feet slightly wider than shoulder width apart and your knees slightly bent.

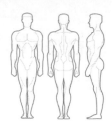

WHAT IT DOES:
Develops cardiovascular conditioning and agility.

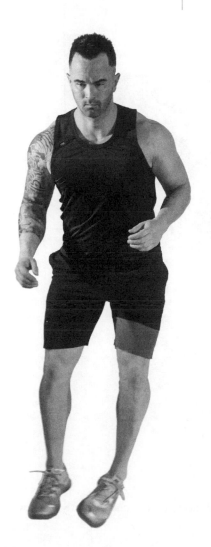

2. Quickly and explosively—with as much force as possible—shuffle on the balls of your feet from side to side, as fast as you can, for the suggested distance and time.

FORM TIP: In order to avoid injury, start slowly, find a rhythm, and then gradually increase the pace.

Short Shuttle **Run**

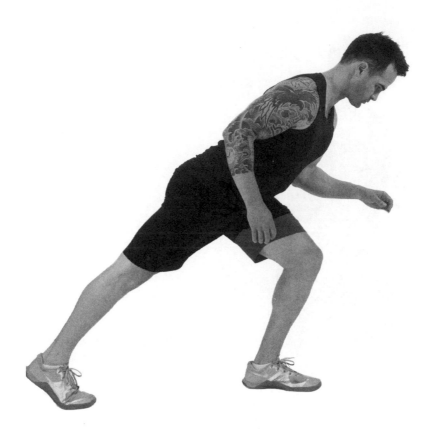

1. Sprint in one direction for the suggested distance.

2. Plant your weight on your outside foot while keeping your knees slightly bent and your hips slightly lowered.

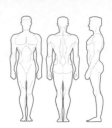

WHAT IT DOES:
Develops cardiovascular
conditioning and agility.

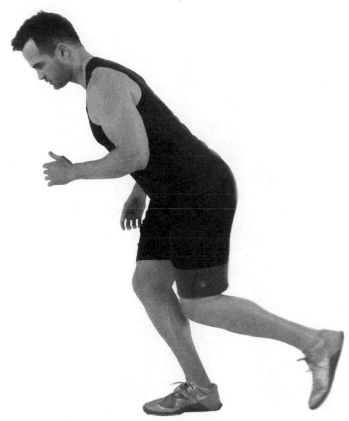

3. Explosively—with as much force as possible—sprint back in the other direction as fast as you can. Continue sprinting back and forth for the suggested amount of time.

FORM TIP: In order to avoid injury, start slowly, find a rhythm, and then gradually increase the pace.

Full-Body **Extension**

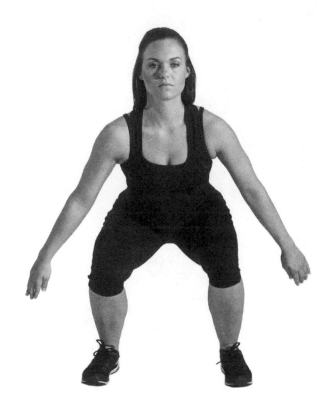

1. Stand with your feet slightly wider than shoulder width apart.

2. Squat down until your thighs are below parallel to the floor, as low as you can comfortably go, swinging your arms behind you.

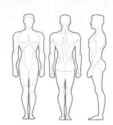

WHAT IT DOES:
Develops cardiovascular conditioning, full-body power, and explosiveness.

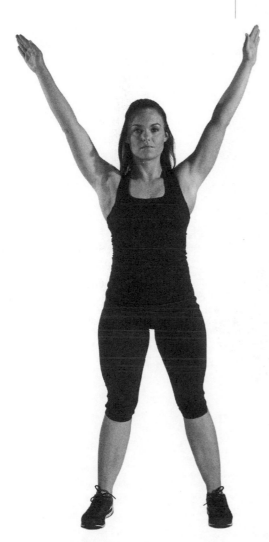

3. Explosively—with as much force as possible—stand back up as fast as you can, reaching your arms as far over your head as you can. Continue squatting up and down, quickly and explosively, for the suggested amount of time.

FORM TIP: To generate as much power as you can during the extension phase, imagine you are tossing something over your head as far as possible behind you.

Full-Body **Band Extension**

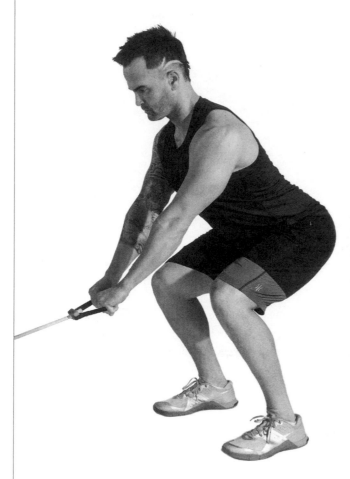

1. Anchor a resistance band to a secure surface (such as a railing or a bedpost) at ground level. Grasp the handle of the band with both hands and step back until the band develops a moderate amount of tension.

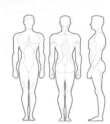

WHAT IT DOES:
Develops cardiovascular conditioning, full-body power, and explosiveness.

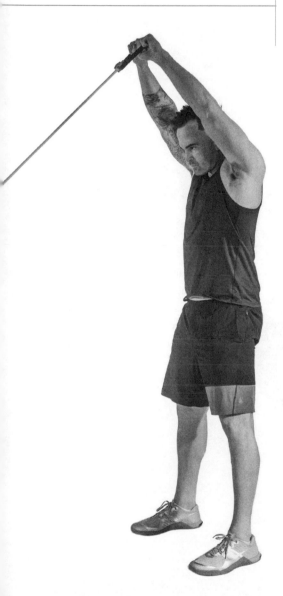

2. Squat down, holding the handle of the band with both arms out in front of you, until your thighs are about parallel to the floor.

3. Explosively—with as much force as possible—stand back up as fast as you can and simulate throwing the band directly over your head. Continue squatting up and down, quickly and explosively, for the suggested amount of time.

FORM TIP: To avoid straining the shoulders, pull the band up only directly above your head and no farther.

Band **Swimmer**

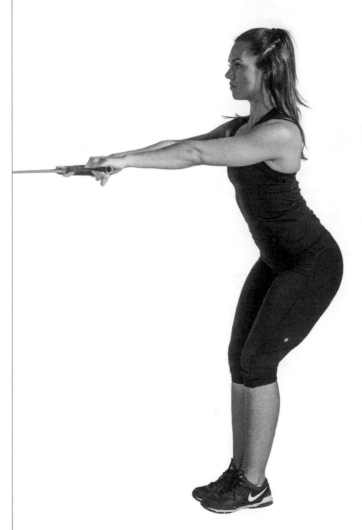

1. Anchor a resistance band to a secure surface (such as a railing or a bedpost) at chest level. Grasp the handles of the band and step back until the band develops a moderate amount of tension.

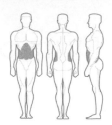

WHAT IT DOES:
Develops cardiovascular conditioning, full-body power, and explosiveness while also strengthening the abdominals.

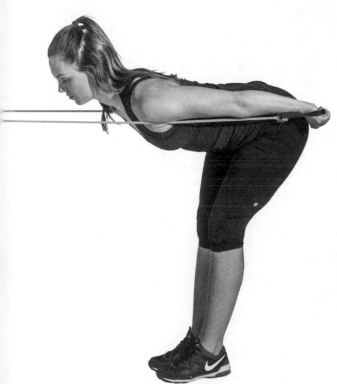

2. Keeping your arms straight out in front of your chest, push your hips back while keeping a slight softness in your knees. Lean forward, pulling your torso forward with your abdominals, while simultaneously driving your straight arms back toward your hips. Think about driving your chest down toward your thighs and pulling your arms to your pockets.

3. Extend back up, allowing your arms to come to chest level. Repeat for the suggested amount of time.

FORM TIP: This is a coordinated movement. If you are having trouble, think "hips back, chest down, arms through."

Dumbbell **Swing**

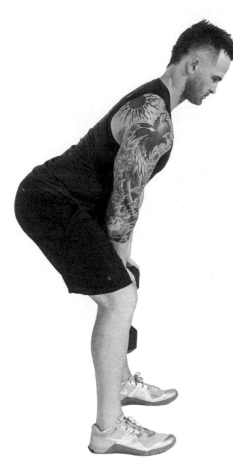

1. Stand with your feet slightly wider than shoulder width apart, arms hanging straight down between your legs, cupping one end of a dumbbell in your fingertips.

WHAT IT DOES:
Develops cardiovascular conditioning, full-body power, and explosiveness and strengthens all the muscles on the back side of your body.

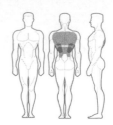

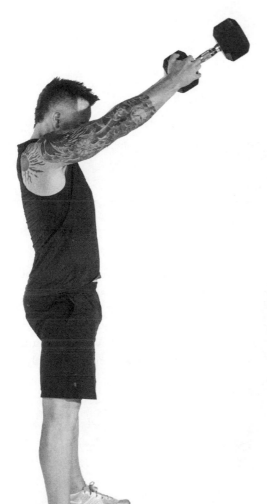

2. Push your hips back and lean slightly forward.

3. Explosively—with as much force as possible—thrust your hips forward and swing the dumbbell to chest level. Repeat for the suggested amount of time.

FORM TIP: Do not bend your knees too much. Think about hinging your hips back and then thrusting them forward. Your hips should be doing 90 percent of the work.

Body Weight **Thruster**

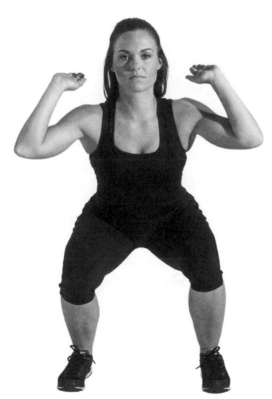

1. Stand with your feet slightly wider than shoulder width apart with your hands at shoulder level, palms facing up. Squat down until your thighs are below parallel to the floor, as low as you can comfortably go.

WHAT IT DOES:
Develops cardiovascular conditioning as well as full-body power and explosiveness.

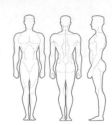

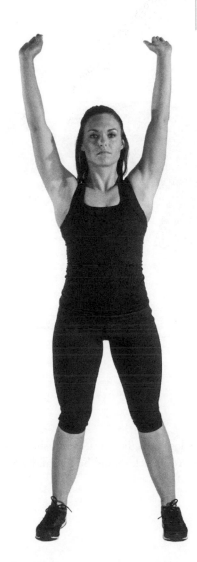

2. Explosively—with as much force as possible—stand back up, straightening your legs and arms while pressing your arms above your head. Repeat for the suggested amount of time.

FORM TIP: To generate as much power as you can while you stand up, imagine you are pushing something over your head as high as possible.

Mountain **Climber**

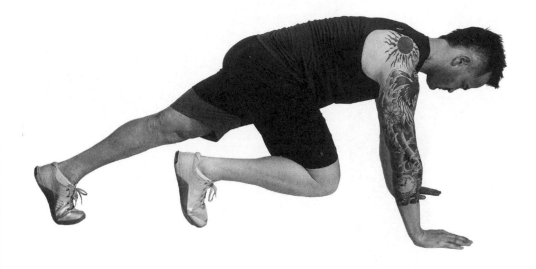

1. Assume a push-up position with your hands on the floor directly beneath your shoulders and your feet shoulder width apart on the balls of your feet. Your back should be flat, and your neck should form a straight line with your back.

WHAT IT DOES:
Develops cardiovascular conditioning, core strength, and shoulder stability.

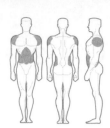

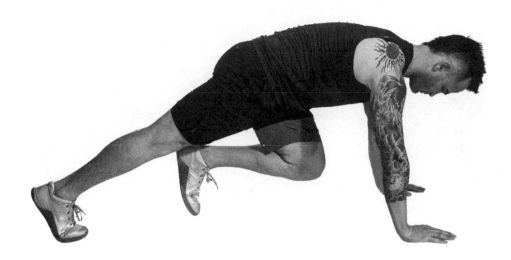

2. Keeping your abdominals tight, vigorously bring your right knee in toward your shoulders, then your left knee.

3. Continue alternating sides in this fashion, not allowing your hips to sag and keeping a steady pace, for the suggested amount of time.

FORM TIP: Focus on driving your legs in and out, fully extending and then flexing your hips, as though you are sprinting.

Cross-Body **Mountain Climber**

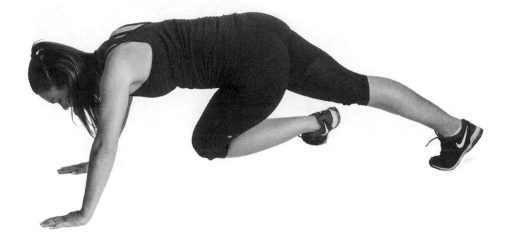

1. Assume a push-up position, with your hands on the floor directly beneath your shoulders and your feet shoulder width apart on the balls of your feet. Your back should be flat, and your neck should form a straight line with your back.

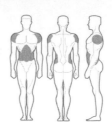

WHAT IT DOES:
Develops cardiovascular conditioning, core strength, and shoulder stability.

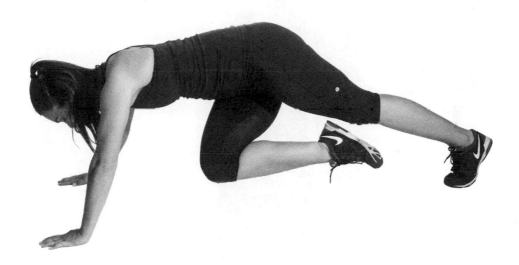

2. Keeping your abdominals tight, vigorously bring your right knee toward your left elbow. Bring your right leg back to the starting position before immediately driving your left knee toward your right elbow. Continue alternating sides in this fashion, not allowing your hips to sag and keeping a steady pace, for the suggested amount of time.

FORM TIP: Exaggerate the "cross-body" motion to fully engage your core and side abdominals. Really think about trying to touch your knee to your elbow.

Jumping **Jacks**

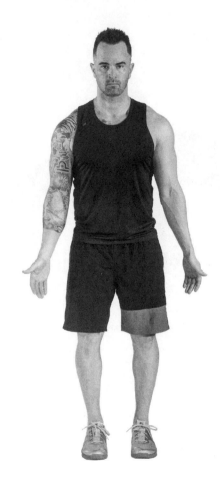

1. Stand in an upright position with your legs together and your arms held straight down to your sides.

2. Get onto the balls of your feet and explosively—with as much force as possible—extend your legs out to the side while simultaneously bringing your arms out and above your head.

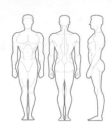

WHAT IT DOES:
Develops cardiovascular conditioning.

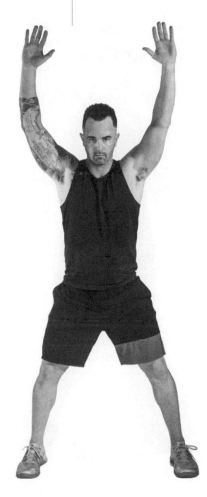

3. Immediately bring your legs back in and your arms back down to your sides. Continue in this fashion, going in and out, for the suggested amount of time.

FORM TIP: Develop as much power and speed as possible when moving your arms and legs in and out.

Body Weight **Prisoner Squat**

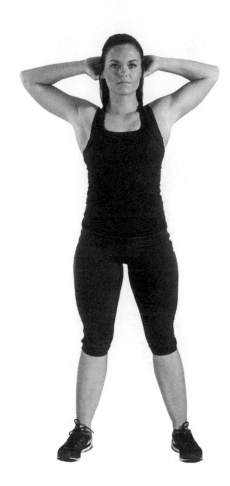

1. Stand with your feet slightly wider than shoulder width apart, with your hands behind your head and your elbows out.

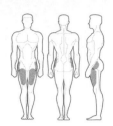

WHAT IT DOES:
Strengthens all the
muscles in your hips
and thighs.

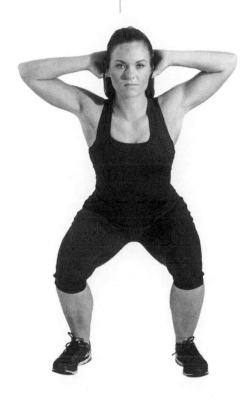

2. Keeping your torso upright and your hands behind your head, push your hips back as you simultaneously bend your knees and squat down until your thighs are below parallel to the floor, as low as you can comfortably go. Make sure your heels stay down and you do not come up onto the balls of your feet.

3. Once you reach the bottom position, immediately stand back to the starting position. Repeat for the suggested number of reps.

FORM TIP: To avoid injuring your knees, do not bounce up out of the squat.

Conclusion
After You Sweat

Once you've completed 9 weeks of the 60-Second Sweat, the logical follow-up questions will be: "What's next? Where do I go from here?" Laying out and detailing exactly what you should do would require another book in and of itself. However, there are certainly some general guidelines and principles I can offer that will point you in the right direction and keep you progressing.

STRENGTH-TRAIN 3 DAYS A WEEK

After you've read this book, the importance of strength training should be engrained in you. Just as it is in the 60-Second Sweat, strength training should be the foundation of your fitness program moving forward. Do a full-body strength-training workout 3 days a week. Despite what some may tell you, setting up a full-body workout is in no way rocket science, nor does it take a great deal of time to execute. All you need is a pressing exercise (which addresses the chest, front of your shoulders, and back of your arms), a pulling exercise (which addresses your back muscles, your rear shoulders, and the front of your arms), a multiple-joint lower-body exercise (which addresses your hips and thighs), and an integrated exercise for your core (which addresses your abdominals and lower back). That's it. Pick just one exercise from each category, and you'll address every muscle in your body—and each workout will take no more than 30 minutes.

Here are the 60-Second exercises that fit into each category:

- **Pressing exercises:** Push-Up, Feet-Elevated Push-Up, Flat Dumbbell Chest Press, Incline Dumbbell Chest Press, Dumbbell Crush Press, Seated Dumbbell Shoulder Press, Dumbbell Push Press, Single-Arm Dumbbell Push Press.
  In addition, you could perform all the dumbbell exercises with a barbell (except the Single-Arm Dumbbell Push Press).

- **Pulling exercises:** Chest-Supported Dumbbell Row, 3-Point Dumbbell Row, Dumbbell Pullover.

  In addition, you could perform chin-ups, pull-ups, lat pulldowns, seated cable rows, and barbell rows.

- **Multiple-joint lower body exercises:** Dumbbell Goblet Squat, Dumbbell Sumo Squat, Dumbbell Front Squat, Rear Foot-Elevated Split Squat, Dumbbell Step-Up, Alternating Goblet Reverse Lunge, Dumbbell Romanian Deadlift.

  In addition, you could perform barbell squats and barbell front squats, leg-press machine, barbell deadlifts, barbell reverse lunges, dumbbell walking lunges, and so on.

- **Integrated core exercises:** Any of the core exercises listed in The 60-Second Sweat exercise index are appropriate. (There are, of course, many other ab exercises out there, but the ones featured in the book are, in my opinion, the safest and most effective, so they should be sufficient to maintain your fitness.)

I recommend 3 to 4 sets of 8 to 12 repetitions for the exercise you choose in each category, resting 60 to 90 seconds between each set. Use the double-progression method: Once you are able to achieve 12 reps of each set of an exercise, increase the resistance slightly and drop back down to the low end of the rep bracket (8 reps). Then build your way back up, adding 1 or 2 reps each set, for each workout, until you once again reach 12 reps on each set. For core exercises, sometimes reps won't apply, since the exercises are timed (think Plank and Side Plank). In these situations, try to perform these types of exercises for more time each workout, never exceeding 90 seconds on any set.

Keep a training log detailing the exercises you did, the number of sets you performed, the number of reps you completed on each set, and the amount of resistance you used on each set. (See page 19 for a blank log form that you can photocopy.) You can put these together in a number of different ways:

- **Straight sets:** Perform a set, rest, and then perform another set of the same exercise until all sets are completed.

- **Paired sets:** Perform a set of one exercise, rest, and then perform a set of a second exercise. Continue in this format until all sets are completed for both exercises.

- **Circuits:** Perform a set of a pressing exercise, followed by a set of a pulling exercise, a set of a multiple-joint lower-body exercise, and a set of an integrated core exercise before starting again with a set of a pressing exercise.

If you choose paired sets, I'd recommend pairing a pressing exercise with a multiple-joint lower-body exercise and pairing pulling exercises with core exercises. If you choose paired sets or a circuit, rest no more than 60 seconds between sets. For straight sets, the rest periods can be up to 90 seconds.

I also advise setting up two separate routines and alternating them. For example, you could create an A workout and a B workout and pick different exercises from the 4 different categories for each workout. For instance, workout A could consist of the Flat Dumbbell Chest Press, 3-Point Dumbbell Row, Dumbbell Goblet Squat, and Side Plank. You would perform that routine, rest a day, and then perform workout B. This could consist of the Incline Dumbbell Chest Press, Chest-Supported Dumbbell Row, Alternating Goblet Reverse Lunge, and Stability Ball Crunch. Then rest another day and perform workout A again, and so on.

How long should you perform the same workouts? There is no hard-and-fast rule here, but generally, I like to run the same workouts for no longer than 6 weeks before substituting new exercises. Many people choose to run the same workouts until they find that progressing becomes difficult (meaning they are not able to add resistance or reps). For some, this may happen after 4 weeks. For others, it's not uncommon to go 10 to 12 weeks before plateauing.

PERFORM HIGH-INTENSITY INTERVAL TRAINING (HIIT) 2 TO 3 DAYS A WEEK

By now you should understand the efficiency and efficacy of HIIT. Coming out of the 60-Second Sweat program, you want to continue to prioritize HIIT. A very easy way to do this? Simply perform 10 to 15 minutes of HIIT immediately after your strength training, using any cardiovascular machines in your gym: treadmills, stationary bikes, elliptical trainers, rowing machines, and so on. Go very hard (9+ on a scale of 1 to 10) for 15 seconds. Then slow down for some low-intensity active recovery for 45 seconds. Repeat this process for 10 to 15 cycles.

What if you don't have access to any cardiovascular equipment? Luckily, the Metabolic Blast circuits detailed in this book are a perfect choice. Another option is to perform 12 to 15 Dumbbell Swings (see page 230) every minute on the minute for 10 minutes. After you perform your swings, take the remainder of the minute to rest before going again at the top of the minute. Repeat 10 times.

If you don't want to—or can't—perform HIIT after your strength training, you can certainly perform it on days off from the weights. So you might do your strength-training workout A on Monday, HIIT on Tuesday, strength-training workout B on Wednesday, another round of HIIT on Thursday, and so on. How to choose, format, and implement HIIT is specific to the individual, his or her time constraints, and life circumstances. The important thing is just to get it in. Because HIIT is by definition intense, it's best if you can rest a day between your HIIT workouts, but if you really need to do them back-to-back because that's when your schedule permits, that's okay.

WALK . . . A LOT

I am a huge proponent of walking. It's easy, can be done anywhere, requires no specialized equipment, and is safe and low impact. It's a perfect way to stay active, burn some calories, and enhance your general health without compromising your recovery from the harder workouts. Walk as much as you can and like. Shoot for 1 to 2 miles every day (you can break this up into smaller chunks). Alternatively, wearing a pedometer—which tracks your steps—or one of the popular Fitbit-like devices is a great way to mindlessly get in more activity. Shoot for 10,000 to 15,000 steps daily.

THE SWIFT SWEAT ROUTINE

So there you have it. Again, these are all very general guidelines, and, without writing another book, I feel that what I've outlined in this section is a very sound and smart plan of attack. You certainly have other options, but I wanted to provide a general template that individuals can tweak for themselves based on their own circumstances.

I want to leave you with one last thing. As I've mentioned several times throughout this book, sometimes life doesn't cooperate, and you literally may have only 10 to 15 minutes to get in a full workout or may not have access to any equipment other than your body weight. If you find yourself in this situation, here is a little "swift sweat" routine you can implement in under 15 minutes. Perform the following as a circuit (all exercises can be found in the exercise index):

- Push-Up Variation (Bench Push-Up, Push-Up, Feet-Elevated Push-Up, and so on): 10 to 15 reps

- Body Weight Prisoner Squat: 15 to 20 reps

- Full-Body Extension: 15 to 20 reps

- Side Plank: 30 per side

- Body Weight Reverse Lunge: 10 reps per side

Go through this circuit, resting only as long as it takes to transition to the next exercise, and follow it as many times as you can in 10 to 15 minutes. Again, this little routine is in no way ideal, but it can be used as a stop gap to get some work in until life settles down and you are able to get back to normal programming. This should be done only when absolutely necessary.

I want to leave you with one final thought: Elite fitness doesn't just happen—it is earned. I have presented you with the most comprehensive, time-efficient, practical, and scientifically up-to-date training program currently available for real-world people like you. I've provided you the road map, but it's up to you to put in the work and to prioritize your health and fitness. Now get sweatin'!

ENDNOTES

1. LaForgia, J., Withers, R.T., and Gore, C.J. (December 2006). Effects of exercise intensity and duration on the excess post-exercise oxygen consumption. *Journal of Sports Sciences,* 24(12), 1247–64.

2. Perry, C.G.R., Heigenhauser, G.J.F., Bonen, A., and Spriet, L.L. (2008). High-intensity aerobic interval training increases fat and carbohydrate metabolic capacities in human skeletal muscle. *Applied Physiology, Nutrition, and Metabolism,* 33(6), 1112–23.

3. Talanian, J.L., Galloway, S.D., Heigenhauser, G.J., Bonen, A., Spriet, L.L. (April 2007). Two weeks of high-intensity aerobic interval training increases the capacity for fat oxidation during exercise in women. *Journal of Applied Physiology,* 102(4), 1439–47.

4. Gillen, J.B., Martin, B.J., MacInnis, M.J., Skelly, L.E., Tarnopolsky, M.A., and Gibala, M.J. (2016). Twelve weeks of sprint interval training improves indices of cardiometabolic health similar to traditional endurance training despite a five-fold lower exercise volume and time commitment. *PLOS ONE,* 11(4): e0154075. doi:10.1371/journal.pone.0154075

5. Daussin, F.N., Zoll, J., Dufour, S.P., Ponsot, E., Lonsdorfer-Wolf, E., Dotreleau, S., Mettauer, B., Piquard, F., Geny, B., and Richard, R. (2008). Effect of interval versus continuous training on cardiorespiratory and mitochondrial functions: relationship to aerobic performance improvements in sedentary subjects. *American Journal of Physiology: Regulatory, Integrative and Comparative Physiology,* 295, (R264–R272).

6. Bartels, M.N., Bourne, G.W., Dwyer, J.H., and Sandel, M.E. (2010). High-intensity exercise for patients in cardiac rehabilitation after myocardial infarction. *PM&R* 2, no. 2: 151–55.

7. Farrar R.E., Mayhew J.L., and Koch A.J. (April 2010). Oxygen cost of kettlebell swings. *Journal of Strength and Conditioning Research.* 24(4), 1034–36.

8. Kokkonen, J., Nelson, A.G., and Cornwell, A. (1998). Acute muscle stretching inhibits maximal strength performance. *Research Quarterly for Exercise and Sport.* 69(4), 411–15.

9. Phillips, S.M., and Van Loon, L.J. (2011). Dietary protein for athletes: from requirements to optimum adaptation. *Journal of Sports Sciences.* 29 Suppl 1:S29–38. doi:10.1080/02640 414.2011.619204

INDEX OF EXERCISES